ConBody

CONBODY

The Revolutionary Bodyweight Prison Boot Camp, Born from an Extraordinary Story of Hope

Coss Marte

with Brandon Sneed

ST. MARTIN'S GRIFFIN 🐾 NEW YORK

CONBODY. Copyright © 2018 by Coss Athletics, LLC. All rights reserved. Printed in the United States of America. For information, address St. Martin's Press, 175 Fifth Avenue, New York, N.Y. 10010.

www.stmartins.com

The Library of Congress Cataloging-in-Publication Data is available upon request.

ISBN 978-1-250-12602-3 (trade paperback)
ISBN 978-1-250-12603-0 (ebook)

Our books may be purchased in bulk for promotional, educational, or business use. Please contact your local bookseller or the Macmillan Corporate and Premium Sales Department at 1-800-221-7945, extension 5442, or by email at MacmillanSpecialMarkets@macmillan.com.

First Edition: March 2018

10 9 8 7

To Jose Lallave, Pilo, Ivan Morillo, Joel Pena,
Sultan Malik, and the whole ConBody team—and, of
course, Mama, Patria Martinez—for your loyalty, for your
hunger, and, most importantly, for your friendship that
has led me through this incredible life.

Run, run, Honey Bun!

—The guys on S-Block, watching me run

Contents

Acknowledgments

I have so many people to thank for this book, for my life. Here are a few:

My mom Patria Martinez, for going so far out of your way to visit me in prison, and for always making sure that I am OK.

My ConBody staff and trainers—Sultan Malik, Ray Acosta, Shane Ennover, Derek Dresher, Chris Kennedy, Serytta Wright for believing in me, and in this, and for pushing us to the next level and making ConBody something that I could scale.

Catherine Hoke and Defy Ventures, and all your staff, for giving me a second chance in life.

Elizabeth Lambos and Michael Mintz, for being great mentors, and for always being there to give me a helping hand.

Scott Graulich, I wouldn't be able to do any of this without you.

Jenn Shaw, for your help.

Cathaniel, for being an incredible son, and the most righteous person I know.

My father Claudio, my brother Christopher, my sisters Claudia and Carolina, for being there for me not just financially when I needed you, but anytime for anything, and for still always asking if I need a helping hand.

Michael and Lauren, my editors at St. Martin's, and all the rest of the St. Martin's team.

My agent, Eric Lupfer at Fletcher & Co.

My coauthor, Brandon Sneed—just write whatever you want for yourself, just maybe not about the first time you worked out with us back in the day and almost passed out.

ConBody

INTRODUCTION

More Than Fitness

If I can go from a fat, dying drug kingpin at twenty-four to a healthy and successful entrepreneur a few years later, then c'mon—there's no fucking way you can't at least get in shape.

The soul of ConBody is simple: Just do the time.

It's hard, especially in the beginning, but there are lots of things that are much harder. Like knowing your kid is growing up with a mother or a father who isn't giving them his or her best—or maybe isn't even there at all. Or getting beaten by guards for looking at them in a way they didn't like. Or when, after they beat you, they write you up for "fighting" them—and then throw you in solitary.

We all do things that land us in prison, in one way or another, sometimes literally, sometimes metaphorically, sometimes both.

Everyone is human. Everyone makes mistakes. Hell, everyone commits crimes. It's just a matter of whether you get caught.

Not that everyone is a drug kingpin, either, of course.

But the point is, people make mistakes, and find themselves imprisoned, literally or figuratively, or both.

First, we have to realize that we did make mistakes. We did something we should not have done, perhaps repeatedly, and our prisons are the consequence of those actions.

Second, we need an opportunity to grow from it. We need to be given the chance to change and to show the world that change is possible.

Even for drug kingpins.

What I want to do with this book is the same thing I want to do with ConBody all around the world: I want to teach you in a way that hopefully helps you learn lessons that took me a lot of pain and suffering to learn first. This book is about more than fitness. It is about the things that lock us up, and the things we can do to be set free.

I've learned that getting locked up isn't actually the worst thing that can happen to us.

The worst thing that can happen is learning what it takes to be free, and then not doing it—not living free when we could.

|||||||||

I've been arrested more than a dozen times in my life.

I've done hard time twice.

I've spent more time than I care to remember at Rikers Island.

I've been a millionaire and lost it all because I made those millions as a drug kingpin.

I'm thirty-one years old now, which is two years older than prison doctors once told me I would live.

I am a father and a son and a brother and a friend.

I'm the creator of ConBody, the "prison-style boot camp" sweeping New York City and taking aim at the rest of the world. I developed it in prison five years ago, after finding ways to work out in my cell so that I could lose enough weight and become healthy enough to save my life.

If that's possible for me, it's definitely possible for you.

That's what this book is about: Giving you a chance to see what's possible for yourself.

Because now, in many different ways, ConBody is my chance to show the world what is possible.

|||||||||

This book will show you the ConBody workout and story, breaking down my journey in a way that helps you along yours.

I'll show you how I got so unhealthy in the first place, which is a lot about how we all become so unhealthy. I went from a star high school soccer and baseball player to someone deathly overweight, all in just a few short years.

I'll show you the very basic, clumsy, awkward ways I got started on the way to losing weight. (Spoiler alert: When I started, I couldn't even do a push-up or a pull-up.)

I'll show you what I did to lose seventy pounds in six months.

I'll show you what I did to keep the weight off.

And along the way, I'll break all the exercises down step by step, with pictures and notes showing what I did and when. These will appear in three separate Tiers:

▼ **Tier 1,** where I started

▼ **Tier 2,** where I ramped things up

▼ **Tier 3,** where I pushed myself as hard as I could

I'll also mix in some workout games I learned, such as:

▼ **Card Game:** going through a whole deck of cards with each suit and value meaning different workouts

▼ **21 Down:** a killer push-up game

▼ **Prison Baseball:** a series of kick-ass supersets

And at the end, I've compiled a three-month ConBody prison boot camp to get you started.

IIIIIIIII

ConBody is designed for anyone and everyone, regardless of whatever shape you are in. Whether you're so out of shape you are literally dying, like I was, or if you're in okay shape, but maybe less healthy than you'd like to be and in need of a jolt. Or if you are already in great shape, but want a fresh new workout that is also ridiculously low maintenance.

These workouts are all bodyweight exercises you can do anywhere, whether in a Manhattan apartment, or a hotel room on the road—or, of course, if you're where I was when I first began, in a prison cell.

The workouts outlined in this book are described exactly as those that I did in prison.

Nothing fancy.

No gimmicks.

No bullshit.

Just workouts born in a prison cell. Workouts that saved my life.

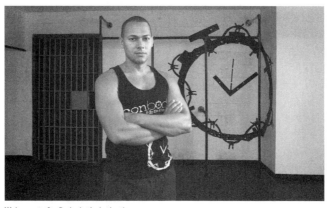

Welcome to ConBody. Let's do the time.

1

LOCKED UP

About a year after I went to Rikers for the second time, the prison doctors told me that I'd probably be dead in five years.

I was only twenty-three.

||||||||

You never *plan* to get fat and so out of shape that it starts killing you, same as you never plan to end up in prison.

You're just living life, trying to make it better, dealing with the pain of it, then things go wrong—something always goes wrong—and the next thing you know, your vices have won and you're in a cell at Rikers and your body feels something like a prison, too.

I'd been to Rikers before, about eight years earlier, and the funny thing about it is that I was in good enough shape back then to literally exercise my way to freedom.

I was seventeen years old and I was running a drug-dealing business based in my home neighborhood, Manhattan's Lower East Side. I'd been dealing drugs since I was thirteen and I'd gotten pretty good at it. Made millions a year. One day the NYPD caught me making a delivery to a crack house, and they found about a dozen bags of cocaine I'd sewn into the lining of my jacket.

I got six years (three in prison, three on parole).

Soon as they let me, I entered "Shock," a boot-camp program that inmates can join if they have three or fewer years left on their sentence and don't have a violent record. Run by f-ing crazy ex-Marines, the idea behind the program is to apparently hammer some discipline into our heads.

Every day, we were up at 5:00 a.m., given just eight minutes to dress, and everything had to be done just the right way—beds made right, clothes worn right, addressing superiors just right: *Yes, sir!* this; *Hoo-ah!* that.

And every day, they made us work out for hours and hours. Jogging, jumping jacks, push-ups, pull-ups, dips, on and on. Many nights, they woke us up in nothing but our boxers and bare feet, even during the winter in the snow. It was brutal and seemed like their idea of helping us was just to torture us for six months—but if you made it through all six months without quitting, then you got to go home.

I was in good shape. I'd played soccer and basketball until my junior year, and I was one of the best players on my high school teams before I quit to focus on my drug business.

I made it through Shock, and it definitely didn't "rehabilitate" me the way they claimed it should. When I first got locked up, I still worked it out to keep running my business from the inside (and even made some money sneaking drugs in for guys who were locked up with me).

And soon as I went home, my boys celebrated by showering me with $10,000 in cash in the middle of Eldridge Street and giving me a new Lincoln Navigator.

That's about when I started getting unhealthy.

‖‖‖‖‖

During that next year, my girlfriend gave birth to my son, "Lil C," and although I knew I wasn't ready for kids, I fell in love with him the second I saw him.

For a minute, I thought that Lil C was helping me settle down. I wanted to be the right kind of dad for him, you know? Take him to Yankees games, not do work that risked taking me away from him, that kind of stuff.

But before long, I was right back out there, hustling more than ever. I never moved anymore. I bought with Joey, my business partner, a brand-new BMW M3 and basically turned it into an office. I drove everywhere—even if I was just meeting someone a hundred feet down the street, I'd drive there instead of walking.

And even then I didn't move, because I usually had someone in the passenger seat working like an assistant who would hop out to handle things.

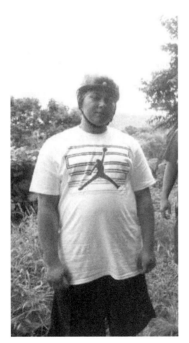

I ate like crap. Nothing but street food.

I drank a lot.

I smoked two packs a day.

And I smoked a lot of weed.

I was living life exactly how I wanted, with no clue that it was killing me.

I don't have many pictures from my old drug kingpin days, but I want you to see me like this, so you know what I looked like at my worst. This picture was taken on a trip to the Dominican Republic not long before I was arrested.

|||||||||

It was March 2009 when the cops busted me again. They'd been trying to get me for years and long story short, they finally did, thanks to a guy I worked with who didn't know they were tracking his cell phone.

Among other charges—organized crime and the like—they charged me as a drug kingpin.

This time I got twelve years.

I spent the first eleven months back at Rikers while I fought the charges. I was still able to get weed—some COs would sell it to me, which is actually pretty common in there—and I still ate like crap, because prison food is almost nothing but crap.

What you see in the movies is what they feed you, if not worse. Mostly we ate sloppy joe–type stuff, and frequently, on especially gross days, some kind of porridge with black seeds in it. I don't really know what it was, only that it came in plastic bags that they boiled and then poured into your pan—and it was gooey and tasted disgusting. No seasoning or anything. We called it "bird food."

Sometimes we got old-school burgers with the thin, flat patties that were okay, but really, the only food we looked forward to was on chicken patty day (though we would call them pigeons, not chickens).

To stay sane, I'd treat myself to the "Prison Burrito."

The Prison Burrito was a custom-made delicacy from items you could only buy at the commissary: ramen noodle soup, cheese rice, Doritos, Slim Jims, maybe some tuna or salmon. Heat the soup and the rice and crumple up the chips, and then dump the soup and rice into the chip bag, mix everything else in there, and boom—Prison Burrito.

So yeah, I was fat and getting fatter.

Still, I had no idea my health was so bad until those prison doctors told me I was basically dying.

||||||||

Before I left Rikers, New York's drug laws changed, and those changes reduced my sentence from twelve years to seven. (Shout-out to Governor David Paterson!)

Fighting my charges didn't work out, though, so they transferred me upstate to Ulster Correctional Facility. The food there wasn't any better, but the doctors gave me a medical exam.

I knew I was fat, and I wasn't exactly surprised when they told me my blood pressure and cholesterol were bad—but then they dropped the bomb: My results were so bad that if I didn't change something, then sometime in the next five years, I would probably die of a heart attack.

I was twenty-four.

||||||||

Soon as I got back to my cell I paced back and forth for a few minutes, then I did some jumping jacks, then I used the side of my bunk to do some push-ups and dips, then I did some sit-ups.

Although really, it's more accurate to say that I tried to do them.

I could barely make it through ten. I counted them off military style, like in Shock: Instead of counting "one, two, three," I counted, "one-two-three-ONE, one-two-three-TWO," making ten reps were really more like twenty . . . but still.

I was dizzy and nauseous and pouring sweat and had to lie down on my bunk.

All I could think was, *I cannot die in this place.*

2

FIRST TWO MONTHS

About Seventy Pounds to Go

At seven o'clock the next morning, I went to the yard and I tried to do some pull-ups.

I couldn't even do one.

Couldn't do dips, either.

I found a bench and used it to do assisted dips.

Then I jogged. I barely made it two laps. About half a mile.

And I felt dead.

||||||||

After a month at Ulster, they transferred me again, this time to Greene Correctional Facility, also in upstate New York, and I stuck with it.

I worked until I was doing a lot of stretches just to make myself move and use my muscles again, plus two sets of twenty-five military counts of these exercises:

▼ Jumping jacks

▼ Calf raises

▼ Dips or assisted dips

▼ Pull-ups (even though I had to get someone to help lift me)

▼ Arm spins

▼ Push-ups superset with gravity push-ups (standing upright, starting with my hands at my shoulders and raising them until my arms were fully extended, bringing them down, then going down to do a push-up)

(I've broken down the above workout after this chapter, starting on page 12, as my Tier 1 workout.)

||||||||||

Eating-wise, I cut out all the junk prison food, and for the first couple of months, I basically lived off canned tuna.

||||||||||

Since we only got four hours a day in the yard, I also worked out all the time in my cell, doing as many jumping jacks and push-ups and dips as I was able.

And when I couldn't do anything else, I just paced two or three steps back and forth, just trying to burn calories.

I wore extra sweatshirts and duct-taped plastic garbage bags to wear over my clothes to make me sweat more, like Bradley Cooper in *Silver Linings Playbook*.

And no matter what, I kept going. When I jogged laps around

the yard, I had to pass another yard on the other side of the fence, the yard for S-Block—troublemakers, guys in partial solitary confinement. Every time I passed their fence, the inmates would swarm to it and mock me. They would yell at me through the fence and bark like dogs.

"Hey, fat dude!"

"Run, Forrest, run!"

"Run, run, Honey Bun!"

All through the first couple of months, I heard so many fat jokes. Some days, they didn't really bother me, but a lot of days they really got to me. Sometimes I wanted to give up.

But I just kept moving, and I didn't react, and didn't let them know they were getting to me. Once they get a reaction from you, they know they have power over you, and it'll only get worse after that.

||||||||

And after two months, I could do twenty to thirty reps per set, and jog about a mile without stopping, and I had lost twenty pounds.

TIER 1
ENTRY-LEVEL WORKOUTS

With these workouts, and with all other workout sections throughout the book, I will make a simple list for you to check off.

If you're confused on how to do the exercises, don't worry: After each list, I have also included photos of every exercise and detailed descriptions of how to perform them.

Stretching

In this general order (military counts of 10–25):

▼ **Neck and shoulder stretch**

▼ **Overhead arm pull**

▼ **Abdominal stretch**

▼ **Chest stretch**

▼ **Upper back stretch**

▼ **Calf stretch toe pull**

▼ **Hamstring stretch (standing)**

▼ **Butterfly stretch**

▼ **Quad stretch (standing)**

▼ **Lower back stretch**

▼ **Knee kisser**

▼ **Groin stretch (standing)**

▼ **Scissor kick**

▼ **Neck rotation**

▼ **Ankle rotation**

▼ Leg swing

▼ Arm swing

Exercise

The first couple of months, I jogged two to four laps at about the length of a standard track, and more if I could hack it, but honestly, I usually couldn't. If it was impossible to go for a run in the yard, I'd run in place in my cell.

In addition, I rotated the following exercises, doing 2 sets of each:

▼ Jumping jack

▼ Calf raise

▼ Standard dip and/or assisted dip (bench dip)

▼ Pull-up (wide/close/regular)

▼ Chin-up (close/wide/regular)

▼ Push-up

▼ Gravity push-up

▼ Arm spin

▼ Sit-up

Some days, I also did laps in between sets. For instance, one set of 25 jumping jacks, then run a lap, then do 25 more, and so on.

TIER 1
EXERCISE PHOTOS

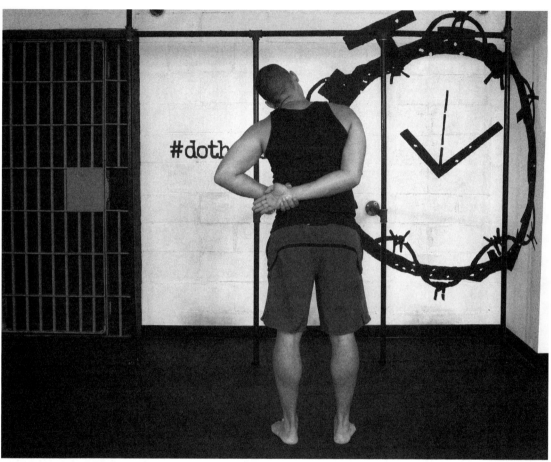

Neck and shoulder stretch.
Place both hands behind your back, on the small of the back. Grab one wrist. Pull that wrist toward the opposite arm. Bring your neck toward the arm, the same direction that the arm is pulling. Make your ear almost touch your shoulder.

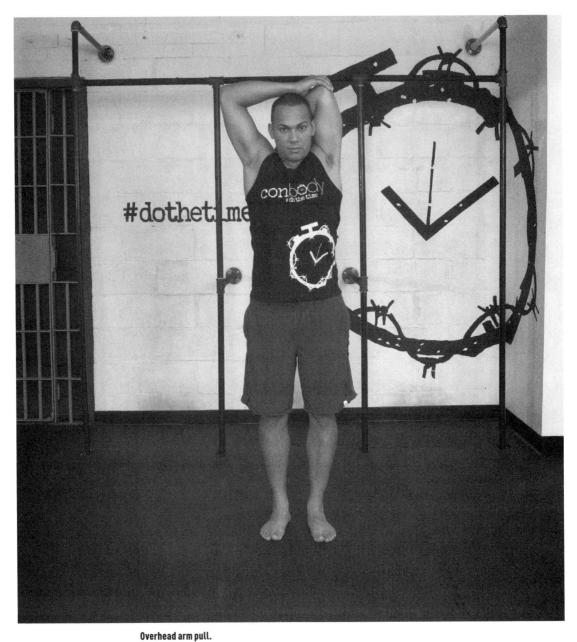

Overhead arm pull.
Put one arm over your back. Use your opposite arm to push down the elbow.

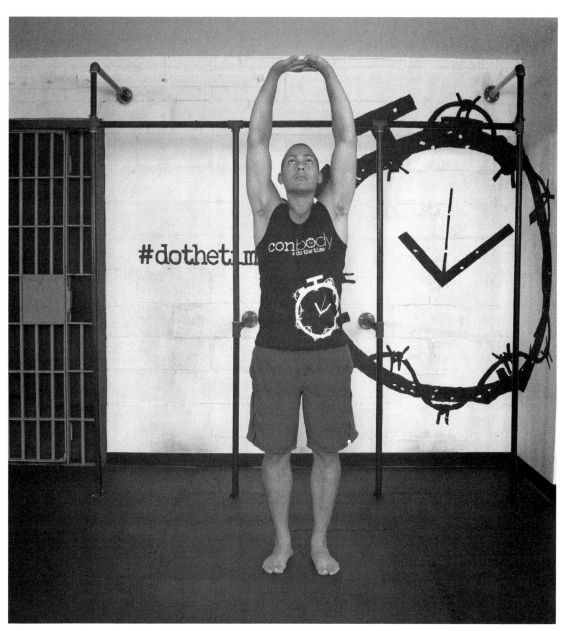

Abdominal stretch.
Interlock your fingers at your chest. Then rotate them upward so your palms face the sky. Try to keep your hands behind your head. Open up your belly.

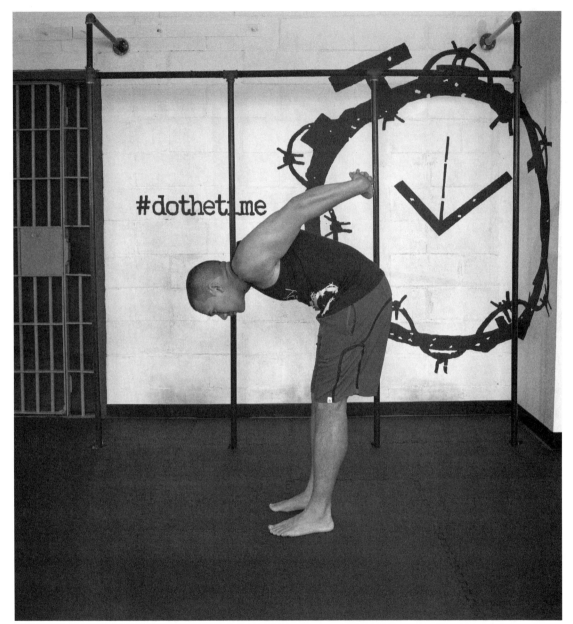

Chest stretch.
Interlock your fingers behind your waist, at the small of your back.
Bend knees slightly. Bend forward.
Flip your hands outward, bringing your arms up.
 Feel your chest stretch.

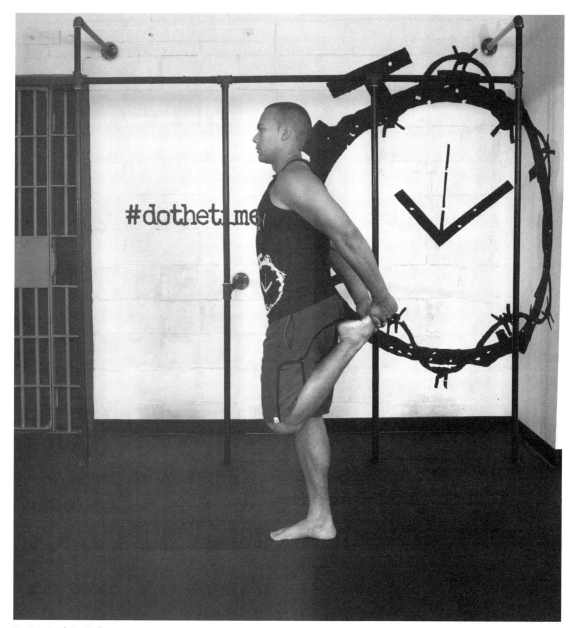

Quad stretch (standing).

Stand up. Stare at one spot to keep your balance. Raise foot toward glute.

Grab foot. Pull foot into glute.

Feel quad muscle stretch in the front of the upper leg.

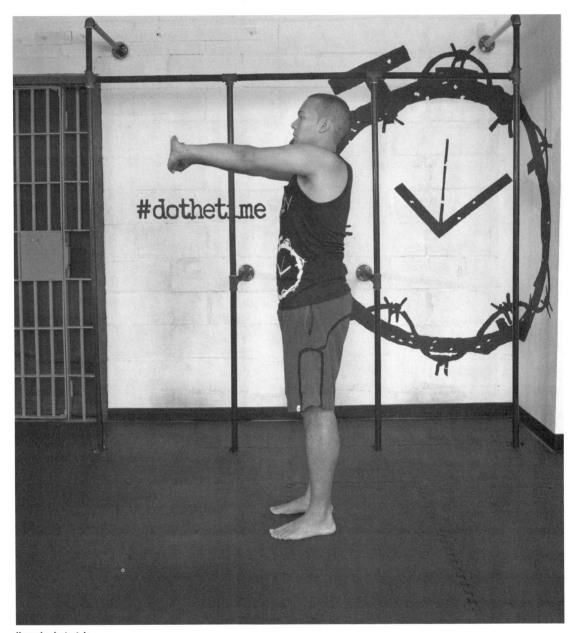

Upper back stretch.

Interlock your fingers on your chest. Stretch them fully extended outward, palms facing away from you.

Curve your back to fully extend your arms forward.

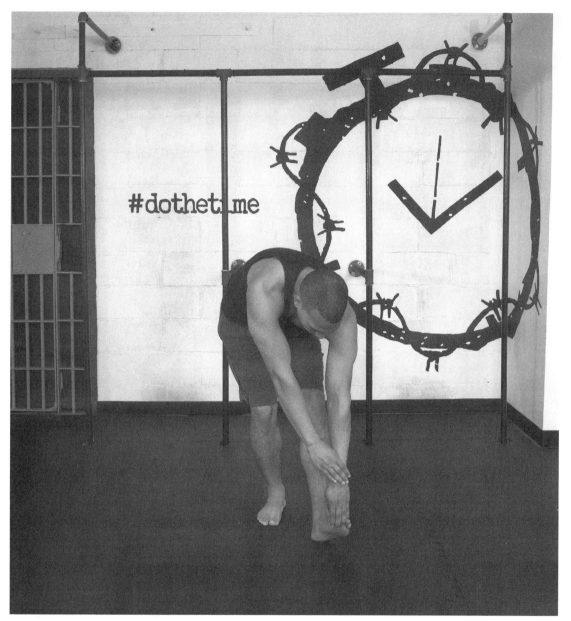

Calf stretch toe pull.

Place your toe up to the sky, heel on the ground. Reach down with both hands to grab that toe.

Bend your opposite knee if you need to.

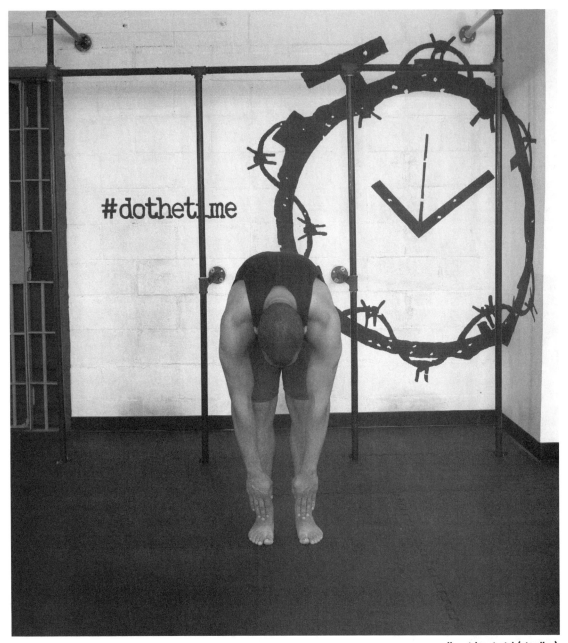

Hamstring stretch (standing).
Put both feet together. Lock your knees.
Reach toward the ground. Try to touch your toes.

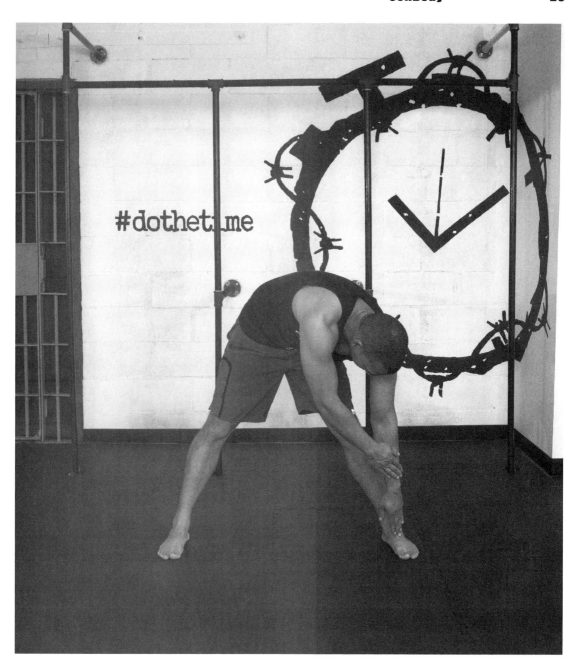

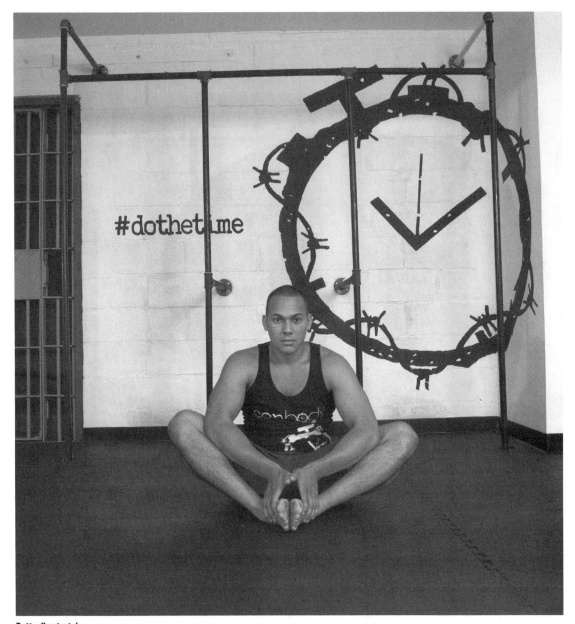

Butterfly stretch.
Put both feet on the ground together sitting down. Grab your ankles. Use your elbows to push down on your knees and open
up your groin area.

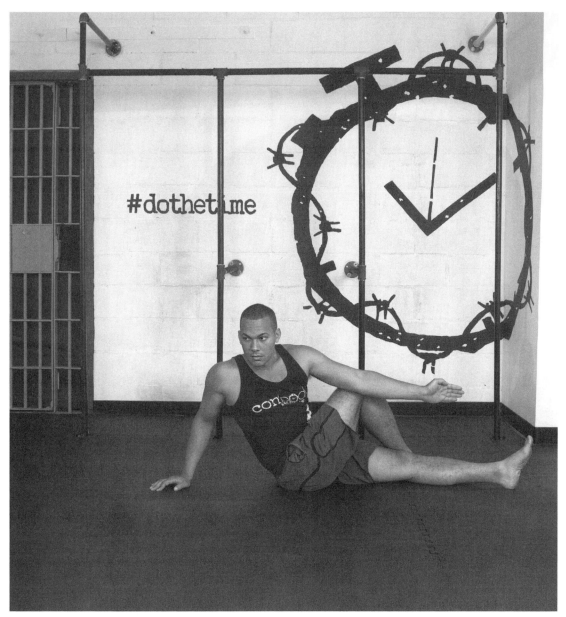

Lower back stretch.
Sit down on the ground. Cross one leg over the other. Bring your opposite arm over your opposite knee looking toward the
wall or in back of you. Twist your body the opposite way. Feel your lower back stretch.

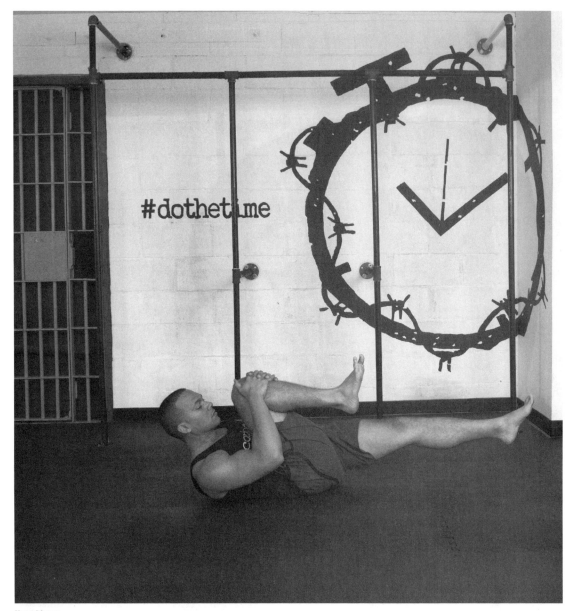

Knee kisser.
Lay flat on back. Grab the knee of one leg. Bring your head toward your knee. Try to kiss your knee.
(Bring your opposite foot off the ground as well.)

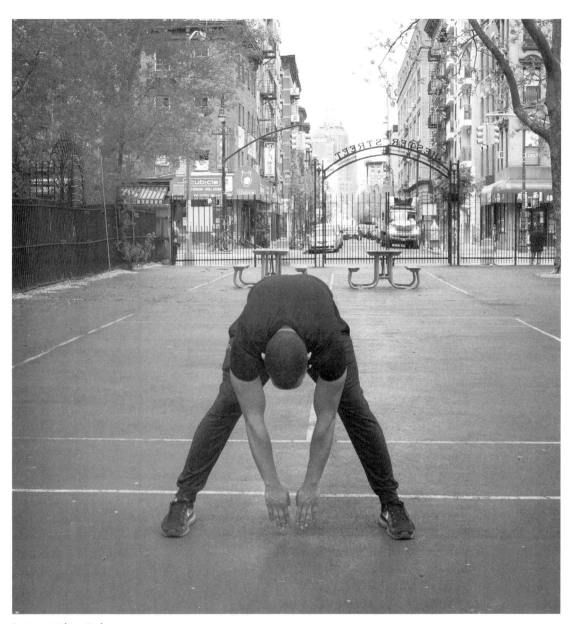

Groin stretch (standing).
Spread legs wide. Reach down to the ground in the middle, and/or lean to one side or the other.

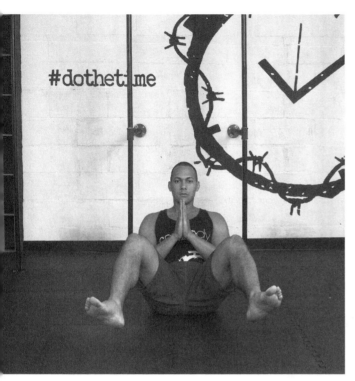 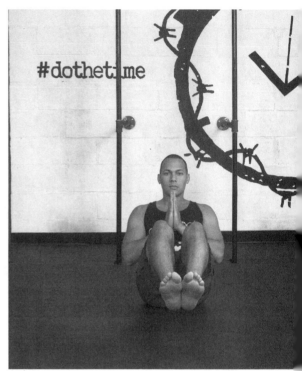

Scissor kick.
Lay flat on back, or sit in reclined position, and keep feet about six inches off the ground.
Spread legs open like scissors, then close. Repeat.

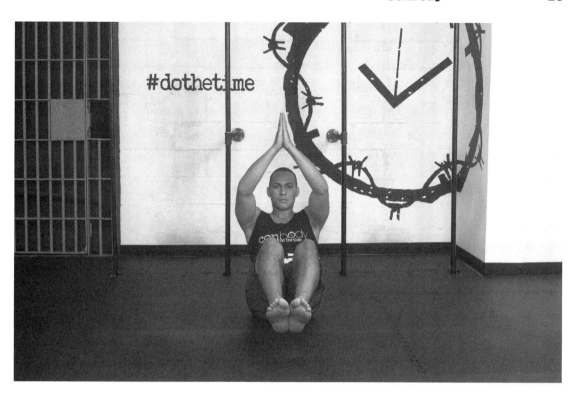

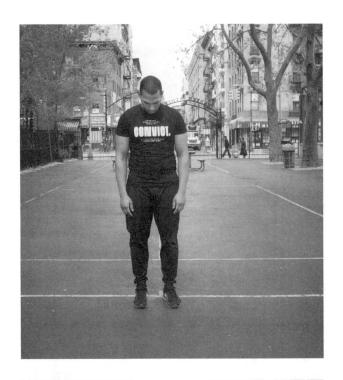

Neck rotation.
Stand up straight.
Rotate head in a big circle
about eight times
in each direction.

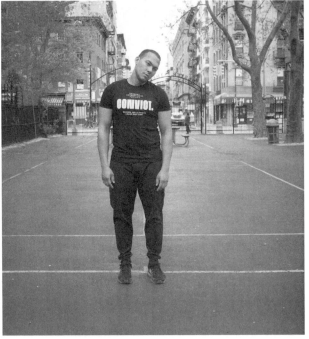

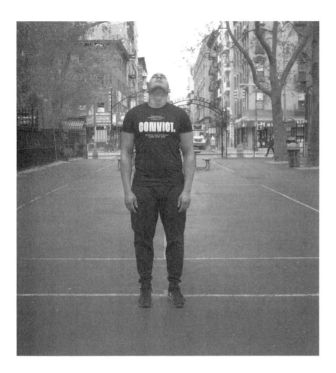

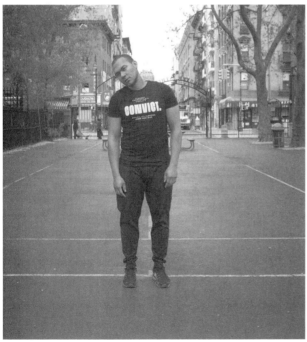

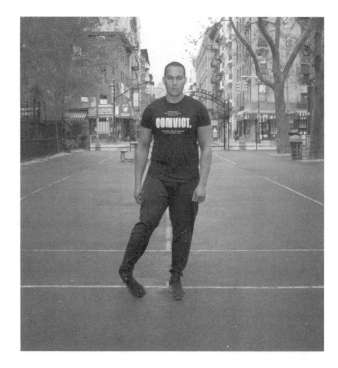

Ankle rotation.
Stand up straight. Put one foot's toe on the ground.
Keep foot loose. Rotate full so ankle stretches.

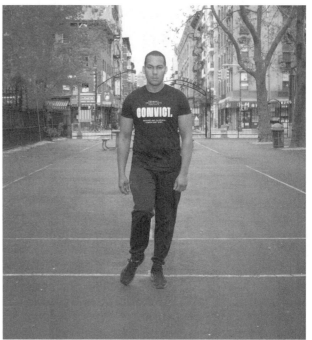

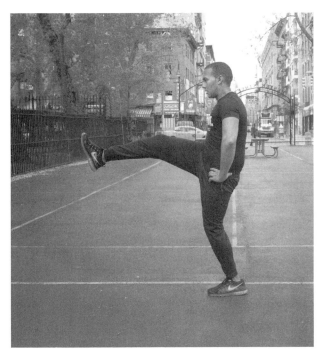

Leg swing.
Lean against wall or something similar for balance if you prefer. Kick one leg all the way forward and up. Then kick back. When you kick back, try to kick your own butt. To do side leg swings: Simply kick leg side to side in front of body. Relax your hip flexors on this and let them open up.

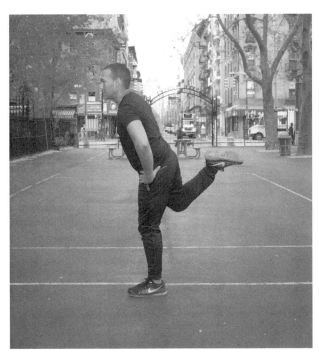

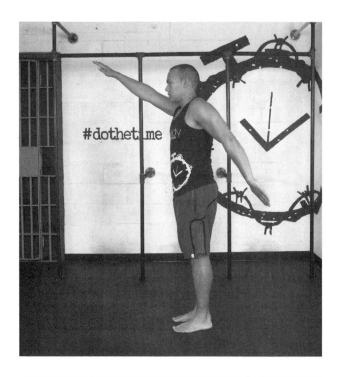

Arm swing.
Put arms to side. Swing them back and forth, one backward, one forward.

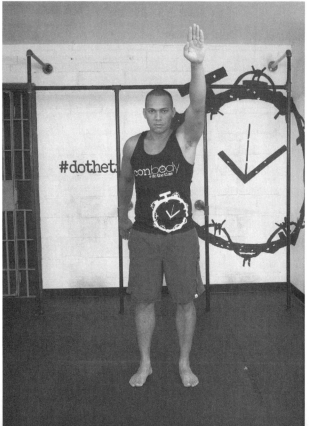

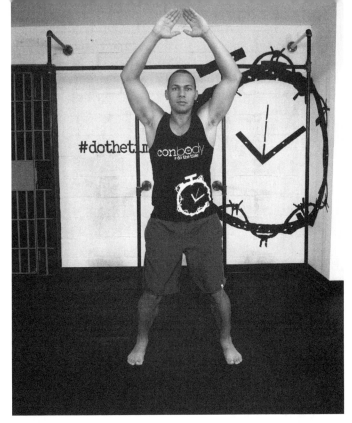

Jumping jack.
Keep your feet together, hands by your side. Jump and spread feet so that you land with your feet shoulder width apart. At the same time, raise hands so that they touch over the top of your head as you land. Jump again, bringing feet together so that they are next to each other when you land. At the same time, bring your hands down to your sides. Repeat quickly.

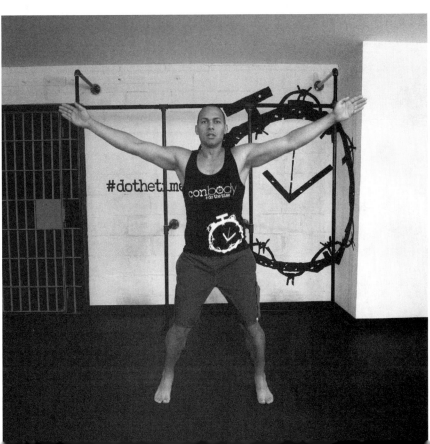

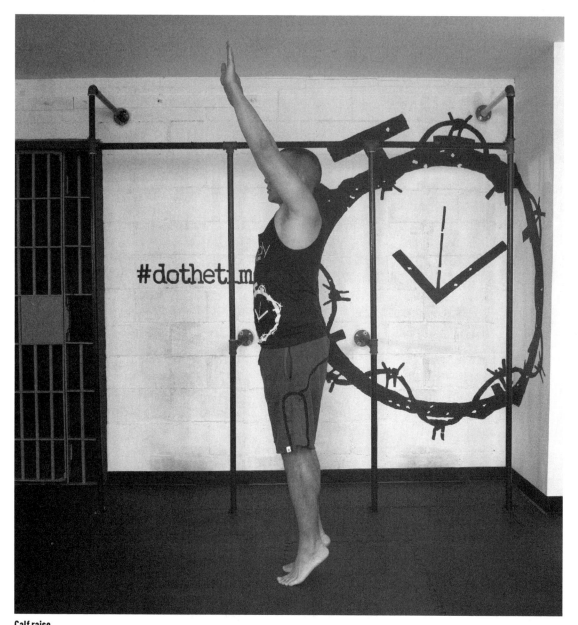

Calf raise.
Stand up straight. Bring your heels up off the ground about five inches. Go up and down.

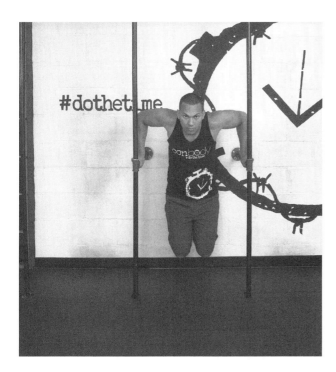

Standard dip.

Place your hands on each side of parallel bars. Push up. Bring your feet off the ground and make your arms straight. This is the starting position. Then dip so that your elbows go down to a 90-degree angle. Keep your feet off the ground. Then push back up.

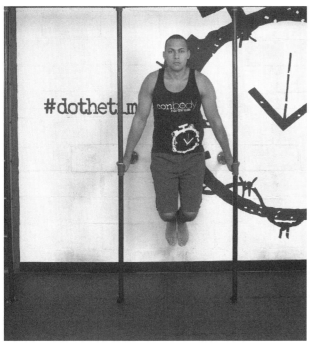

Assisted dip (bench dip).
Use something like a chair, bench,
or ledge. Sit on it.
Bring your butt off the ledge,
to the side. Keep your hands on
the edge of the surface. Bring your
arms to a 90-degree angle as you
dip down. Your butt should almost
touch the ground but not quite. Then
push yourself back up.

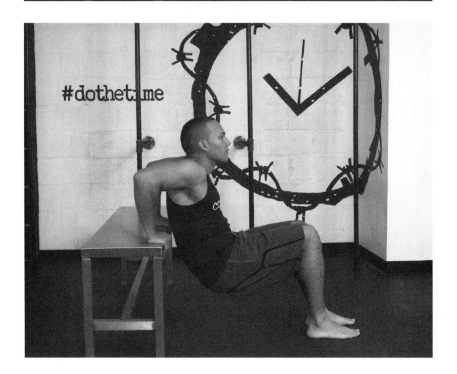

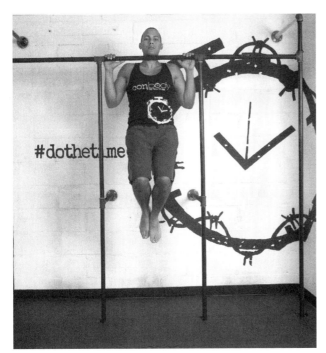

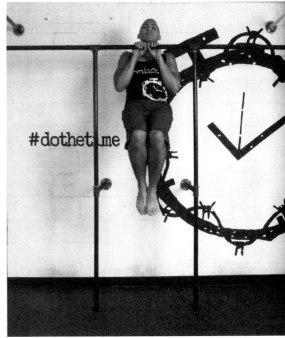

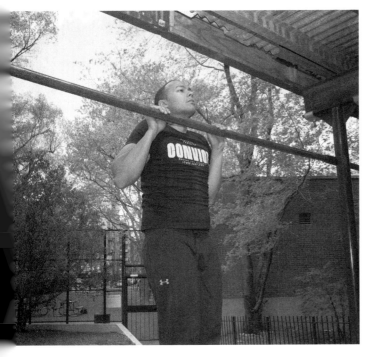

Pull-up (wide/close/regular).
Grab the pull-up bar at shoulder width, palms facing away from you. Thumbs either wrapped around the bar or tucked under the bar. Pull yourself up until your chin goes past the bar. Lower yourself until your arms are straight. Repeat. Beginners: I recommend practicing by doing one pull-up and then holding for 10 seconds. Build up to doing more reps.

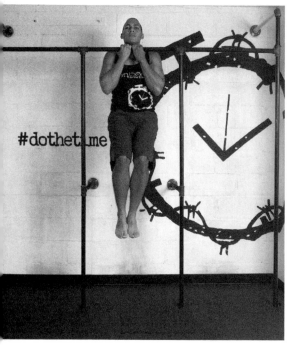
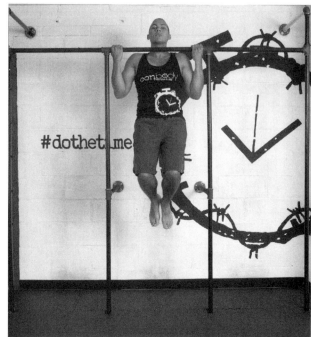

**Chin-up
(close/wide/regular).**
Same as a pull-up, except instead of grabbing the bar
with your palms facing away, grab
with your palms facing yourself.

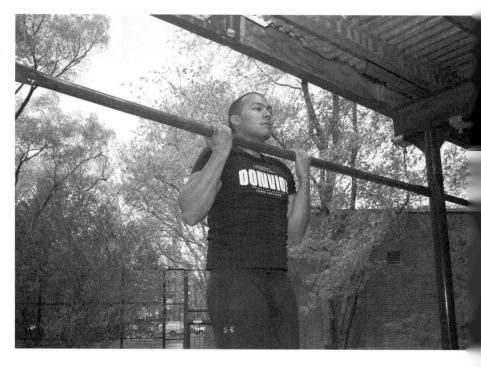

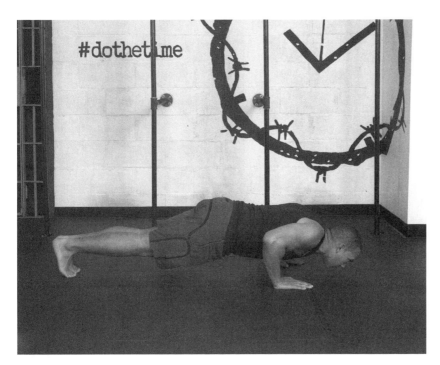

Push-up.
Lay down belly on the ground. Place your hands at your shoulders. Position your arms so that your elbows are at roughly a 90-degree angle and tucked against your side. Push up.
Your entire body should leave the ground. Keep your back flat. Keep your elbows tucked in to your sides instead of letting them spread out sideways. Go up and down, chest to the ground, then back up.

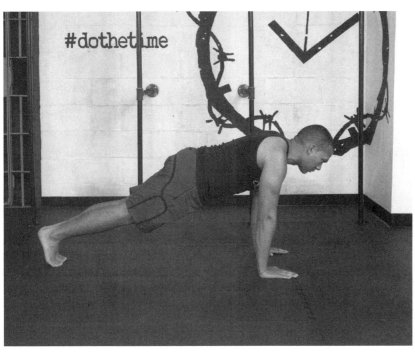

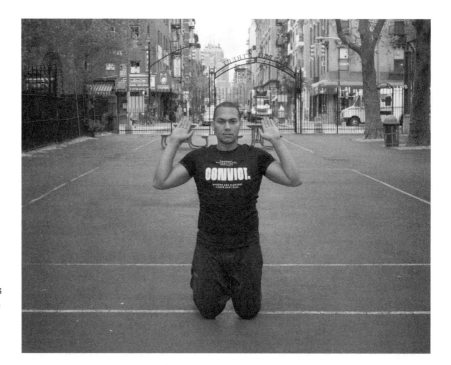

Gravity push-up.
On your knees. Place your hands directly over your shoulders, palms facing the sky. Push up against the air. Fully extend arms. Then bring hands back down to shoulders. Repeat.

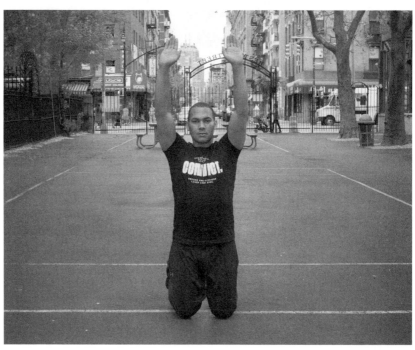

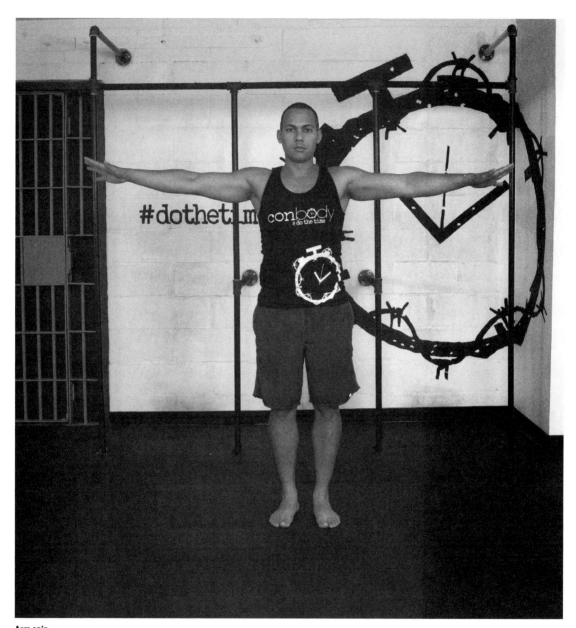

Arm spin.
Fully extend arms to your sides, and do small circles to the front. When rotating them backward, place your palms facing up
to the sky and rotate them backward. Fully extended, keep elbows locked.

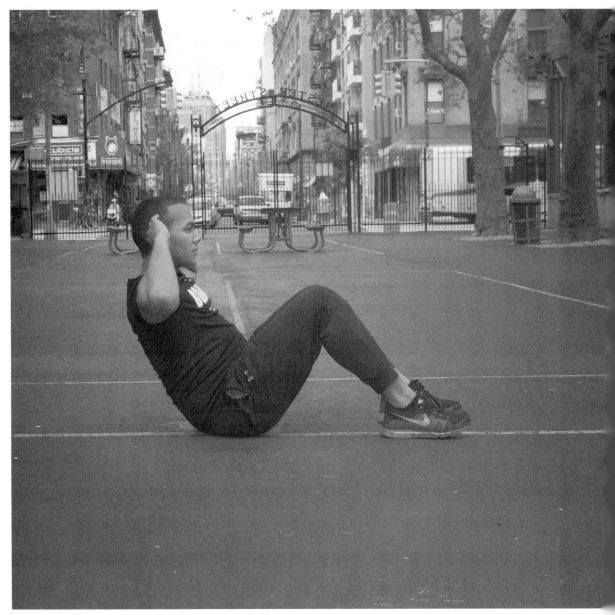

Sit-up.
Sit down. Lie with your back flat to the ground. Tuck your feet back so your knees are up. Place your hands at your temples.
Crunch up until your elbows touch your knees. (Do not lock them behind your head—this tends to make people pull against
the back of their skull, which puts strain on the neck and the spine.)

CONVICT DIET

Eating right was tough in prison because everything from the commissary was processed canned food, or at least that's how I remember it. I found a recent prison menu and it sounds way better than what we had. They're getting kosher food and fresh fruit and vegetable juice and lima beans and all kinds of healthy shit. I wasn't exaggerating earlier when I said that what we got was like what you see in movies. Sloppy joes, that nasty "bird food" porridge with black seeds in it, shitty thin burgers, pigeon patties—I mean, chicken patties.

Prison Burritos saved my sanity for a while, but when it turned out they were also probably killing me, I had to cut them out.

Not gonna lie, it was a struggle to want to keep eating right. I confess that I might've sneaked a Prison Burrito here and there. You gotta stay sane somehow. Below is the recipe for my Prison Burrito:

▼ **Ingredients**

1 pack ramen noodle soup, flavor of choice

1 pack cheese rice

1 bag Doritos

3–4 Slim Jims

1–2 cans tuna or salmon (optional)

▼ **Directions**

Heat soup

Cook rice

Crush bag of Doritos

Dump Doritos into soup

> Dump rice into Doritos bag
>
> Dump soup into Doritos bag
>
> Tear up Slim Jims, dump into Doritos bag
>
> Dump tuna or salmon into Doritos bag (optional)
>
> Mix

Once I decided that I wanted to live past the age of thirty, I tried to eat right.

I cut out lots of carbs and all sauces. That was one of the worst parts—the doctor said I should lay off the sauce stuff, which, when it came to prison chow, was the true good shit. Here's what I tried to eliminate from my diet:

▼ **Bread**

▼ **Processed sugar**

▼ **Juice (Kool-Aid, etc.)**

▼ **Pasta**

▼ **Rice (except for a special occasion)**

▼ **Sauces**

▼ **Gravy**

▼ **Casseroles**

My new diet was mostly pescatarian:

▼ **Fruits (especially apples and boiled plantains)**

▼ **Vegetables (especially potatoes and apples)**

▼ Salmon

▼ Crab in a can

▼ Tuna

▼ Sardines

▼ Calamari

▼ Octopus

▼ Turkey

▼ Canned chicken breast

Thankfully, my family looked out for me, sending me a good amount of food every month. I'd cook all of it. Sometimes I used the microwave, but it was always being used or was busted, so mostly I used a hot pot I rigged up. Hot pots are these small electric burners that come with a small, flimsy plastic "pot" for us to make coffee. I'd take the plastic part off and stick a big Maxwell House coffee can on there and mixed it together. Then I'd rig the wires from the hot pot and line the base of the can with oil and vinegar and onions, then throw stuff in there.

And voilà—sautée.

I'd get some food from chow hall, but usually I tried to cook a bunch for dinner and eat leftovers for lunch the next day.

Oh, and one more thing: Jack Mack. Precooked mackerel in a can, like canned tuna. Its skin is basically just fucking slime and sometimes you'll open a can to find other innards swimming around with the good parts. And it smells like fish ass.

Here's a look at a basic weekly menu of what I tried to eat then, which is basically how I eat nowadays, too:

Monday

▼ **Breakfast**

Orange

Apple

Fish filet

Oatmeal with peanut butter and banana

▼ **Lunch**

Chicken

Mashed potatoes

Mixed vegetables

▼ **Dinner**

Fish

Small amount of rice

Jack Mack

Tuesday

▼ **Breakfast**

Bran flakes

Apple

Orange

Turkey cutlet

Mixed vegetables

▼ **Lunch**

Leftovers from Monday's dinner

▼ **Dinner**

Boiled plantains

Calamari

Cooked broccoli

Wednesday

▼ **Breakfast**

Bran flakes

Orange

Banana

Carrots

Apple

▼ **Lunch**

Leftovers from Tuesday's dinner

▼ **Dinner**

Potatoes

Salmon

Canned collard greens

Thursday

▼ **Breakfast**

Orange

Banana

Oatmeal with peanut butter and banana

Mixed vegetables

▼ **Lunch**

Leftovers from Wednesday's dinner

▼ **Dinner**

Rice

Beans

Tuna

Friday

▼ **Breakfast**

Orange

Apple

Peas

Lima beans

Bran flakes

▼ **Lunch**

Leftovers from Thursday's dinner

▼ **Dinner**

Yuca with sautéed onions

Octopus

Sautéed lima beans from chow hall

Saturday

▼ **Breakfast**

Apple

Orange

Tuna salad

Oatmeal with peanut butter and banana

▼ **Lunch**

Leftovers from Friday's dinner

▼ **Dinner**

Sweet potatoes

Sardines

String beans

Sunday

▼ **Breakfast**

Bran cereal

Apple

▼ **Lunch**

Leftovers from Saturday's dinner

▼ **Dinner**

Chicken

Potatoes

Mixed vegetables

3

MONTH THREE

About Fifty Pounds to Go

After the first couple of months and the first twenty pounds, I began adding and mixing and matching and even inventing lots of different exercises, especially for my legs and my core.

For one thing, I knew that it helped me get in better shape to mix things up like that—you want to keep your body guessing and constantly push it in new and unique ways.

For another, I'm just wired to always push myself harder in everything I do—for better or worse, I always want to go all-out; to go as far as I can. This can be equally powerful for good and for bad.

Going all out and pushing myself to go as far as I could back home is, after all, a big reason why I got into this mess in the first place. That's also why I planned to go right back to dealing again when I got out. I wanted nobody and nothing to be able to stop me.

|||||||||

I based my drug empire out of the Lower East Side in Manhattan because that's where I grew up, a block from Chinatown.

We were poor. My parents had to save for months to get here

from the Dominican Republic. I was still in my mother's womb when they came to America; she was six months pregnant.

We lived in a tiny apartment in a ragged building on Rivington Street. My father ran a bodega and drove a cab, and my mom worked in a factory. I would go with her and sit at her feet.

I made good grades, and I was a good son. But ever since I was eight years old, though, I wanted more. It seemed like every kid in my building, all my cousins and friends, had video game systems—Ataris and Nintendos—and new clothes and shoes, instead of old secondhand stuff like mine. I wanted what they had, so I went door-to-door with a big black trash bag every Sunday night to collect empty beer cans and liquor bottles.

I dreamed about making it big as a pro athlete in soccer or baseball and getting rich off of that. Starting from as young as I can remember, I was always playing soccer and baseball at Roosevelt Park across the block from our building. I loved playing. I loved diving for balls, even on the gravel at Roosevelt.

IIIIIIIII

First time I smoked weed, I was eleven. I was on the roof of my building with my older cousin. I loved the way the weed made me feel—but more than that, I loved the way it felt when people started paying me for it. I was the first kid in my class to smoke weed and when people found out they asked me how they could get some, too.

I made my first drug deal when I was thirteen. Kids in my middle school class found out I smoked and asked how they could get some, so I saved up a hundred bucks and bought an ounce from my cousin. Flipped it for $300. Easiest $200 of my life.

I still dreamed of making the Yankees, but I was done collecting bottles and cans for nickels—to make money in the meantime I became a weed dealer.

A few months later, I started selling cocaine, too. I didn't even have a scale—I bought an eight ball and got some little plastic baggies and just made the bags look right. Made $300 off that.

Within a year I was making $100 a day.

Before long I added ecstasy to my menu and made even more.

I didn't think of selling drugs as a bad thing—it was just something I'd grown up watching a lot of friends do and I thought of it as just another way to make money. Just another job, you know?

And this job, I was good at. I got arrested a bunch but only for little stuff, a tiny bit of weed here and there, nothing serious. I knew how to divvy out my load and hide my stashes.

I never planned to make it some big thing. I was an honor student in school and loved education—and I still loved soccer and baseball, too. I loved running fast and making crazy plays, a striker in soccer and usually playing center field or second base in baseball. Sometimes my name made the paper and I'd keep on dreaming about playing for the Yankees one day.

||||||||

In my sophomore year, a nice boarding school in Rhode Island gave me a scholarship, and I went because my goal in life was to make a lot of money, and I thought that going to school with rich people might teach me something. Maybe I could find some sort of secret.

Instead, I learned that rich people loved drugs just as much as the poor people on my block back home—and they had a lot more money to spend on them. I went right back into business and I made more money from them than I ever had.

That lasted until someone in charge found ecstasy and weed in my room, and they kicked me out and had me arrested. The judge gave me the choice to either fight the charges or to go to rehab for thirty days. That choice was obvious.

And rehab didn't do anything for me except teach me how to be a better drug dealer—a guy I met in rehab taught me how to cook cocaine into crack.

||||||||

When I got back home, I quit soccer and baseball. I'd done the math: Making it in pro soccer or being able to play baseball for the Yankees would take years and years of hard work—and *still* require luck along the lines of winning the lottery. Meanwhile, I could make *more* selling drugs right *now*.

So I quit playing sports. Killed my dream.

My parents and sisters begged me to do life "the right way," but "the right way" felt ridiculous to me. I even judged my sisters and others for taking that path. Working for someone else, making way less money than them to make money *for* them, being stuck and dependent on someone else for your quality of life—no thank you.

I already knew how to make a living, and not just that, but live like a king. I already was my own boss. Like most teenagers, I thought I knew everything and decided that the rest of the world couldn't handle my brilliance.

But I did love my family, and I knew there were ways to be your own boss legally, of course, and I *did* like school and loved—still love—to learn, so I took one more swing at "the right way," finishing high school and going to SUNY-Albany.

But in college, it was like all anyone really cared about was partying, and I loved a good party and I knew how to make parties great (for the right price), and business just kept booming.

They kicked me out after just one semester, and it was back to dealing full-time.

I thought the concept of there being "a right way" to do life was the same as any other religion—same as the concept of God: Most of my family were devout Roman Catholics, but God always felt like a hoax to me.

I had my own scripture: Biggie, in "Things Done Changed":

||||||||

If I wasn't in the rap game
I'd probably have a key knee-deep in the crack game.

||||||||

That was my way.
That was my religion. And in it, I was a saint.
I said fuck knee-deep, and went in to my neck.

||||||||

I missed playing soccer and baseball, and I missed class, but I still hung around Roosevelt all the time, where I might not play sports anymore, but I did sell a whole lot of drugs. One of my main partners-in-crime was my boy Pilo, one of my best friends since we were kids.

I spent most of my time there and hanging around a bodega on my block on the corner of Eldridge and Broome.

Before long, I was making around $3,000 a day. My main menu options were weed, coke, crack, and ecstasy.

Then a fellow dealer friend of mine who had a huge network told me he was "retiring" and asked if I wanted to take over his business.

And from there, I became a millionaire.

I never slept except for taking twenty-minute power naps here and there.

And we partied as hard as we worked, living like we were bigger than rock stars.

I bought everything I ever wanted and bought my friends everything they ever wanted, too. Jordans, clothes, cars, all the best; name-brand everything.

I pimped out a 1993 Fleetwood Cadillac with twenty-two-inch gold rims and ran red lights and parked on sidewalks.

I flew my crew to the Dominican and Puerto Rico on whims.

Just for a fun side hustle we organized a fight club and made money betting on the fighters.

We would hire those Central Park horse-carriage drivers to haul us all over the city. We even gave one of them weed and had him take us through the only McDonald's drive-through in Manhattan—we got the horse an apple pie.

And I became a drug-dealing innovator, doing things nobody in my hood had ever done.

I rigged various buildings on the block to serve as gigantic drug-vending machines: I turned trash chutes into makeshift drive-through windows. One of my boys on the ground would take orders.

One ounce of weed, $200.

Would you like a side of crack with that?

Then he'd call up to the roof, where another one of my guys would then drop a bucket on a line, reel up the cash, then send the product back down.

I modified mailboxes and stairwells to pop open and slide in and out of the wall to secure stashes. Police raids never found them.

I networked with other dealers around the neighborhood and I set up a delivery service. I printed ten thousand business cards and called my business "Happy Endings" after a bar where we always hung out. *We Deliver 24/7. All customers always satisfied.*

I bought my delivery guys bikes and then rented them cars, switching them out all the time to keep the cops guessing.

I put my delivery guys in suits and ties because that way they looked like businessmen and cops don't stop and frisk guys wearing suits. We started focusing our marketing efforts on a key demographic nobody else in my hood ever had: rich, white Wall Street types with loads of cash. People on the Lower East Side came to call me Coss the Boss—sometimes, Coss the *Motherfucking* Boss.

It got to where we were burning through a kilo of cocaine every couple of weeks.

We were like old-school newspaper boys. *Extra! Extra! We got blow!*

ΙΙΙΙΙΙΙΙ

So while trying to lose weight and get healthy in prison, I applied that same instinct to push things to the extreme in my workouts.

I tried to remember what we'd done in the Shock program, and customized those exercises by blending them with some of the ones I was already doing, and created a lot of my own.

I made a list and pulled enough from it each day to do about five sets of upper body five days a week and legs one day a week. (You can see photos of the exercises, starting on page 62.)

I also started using the "Card Game"—each card in a deck represents a certain exercise, with each type of card meaning a certain number of reps. I've broken the exercise down on page 84.

Basically, my whole goal was to confuse my body as much as possible. That way, I made it feel like it was working harder than it actually was—I wanted to make it feel like I had done a thousand push-ups or squats or crunches even if I hadn't.

And along the way, I kept a strict diet. I did let myself eat more than just canned tuna, but tried to eat as healthy as I could. I break that diet down at the end of chapter two, on page 47. (*And since I've gotten out, I have expanded my diet a little more. It's amazing how good healthy food can taste after spending years trying to eat healthy in prison.*)

As a result, by the end of that third month, I lost twenty more pounds for a total of forty.

TIER 2
NEXT-LEVEL WORKOUTS

I ramped up my workouts a lot:

▼ **5 sets of upper body, 5 days per week**

▼ **5 sets of lower body, 1 day a week**

▼ **5 sets of core, 6 days per week**

In addition to Tier 1 (page 12), I started mixing in the following moves. For your convenience, the exercises are provided here first in list form, and then followed by photos with captions that explain how to do them.

Core

▼ **Crab walk**

▼ **One-leg plank**

▼ **Lay-up-and-down**

▼ **Supine bicycle**

▼ **Engine**

▼ **Side-by-side twist**

▼ **Flutter kick**

▼ Windshield wiper

▼ Scissor kick up-and-down

▼ Sit-up

▼ Crunch

▼ Plank

▼ Side leg raise

Other/Full Body

▼ T-bone

▼ Toe touch

▼ Back and forth

▼ Squat jack

▼ Up-and-down

TIER 2
EXERCISE PHOTOS

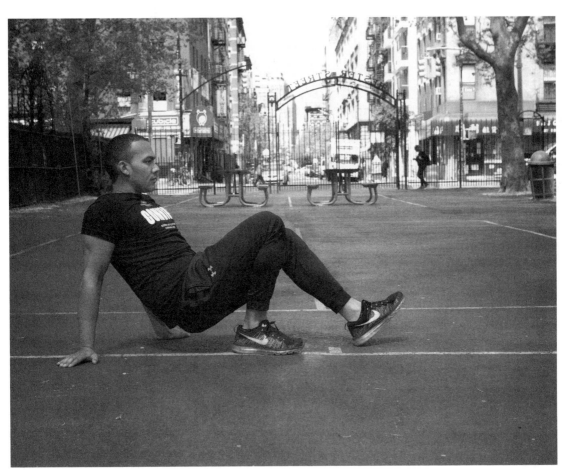

Crab walk.
Sitting down, bring butt off the ground, then hands directly behind your back.
Move forward, same arm at the same time as the same leg
(i.e., right leg moving forward with right arm).
Stay on heels and hands, keeping your butt off the ground.

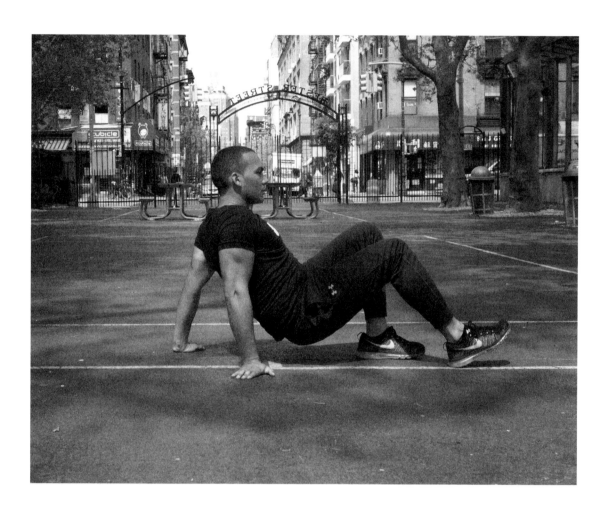

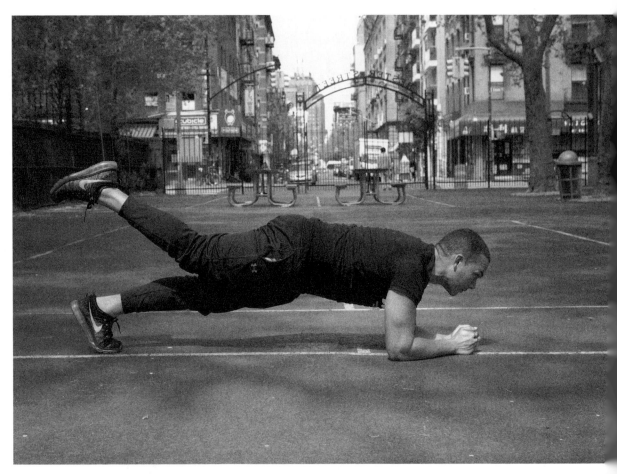

One-leg plank.
Get down on elbows. Do a regular plank. Bring one leg up. Leave your opposite leg on the ground.

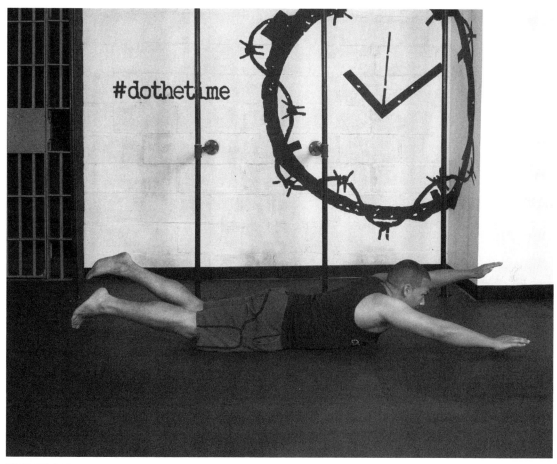

Lay-up-and-down.

Lie flat on the ground, on your chest. Bring your hands and knees off the ground.

Raise them up high as you can and then back down—but don't let them touch the ground.

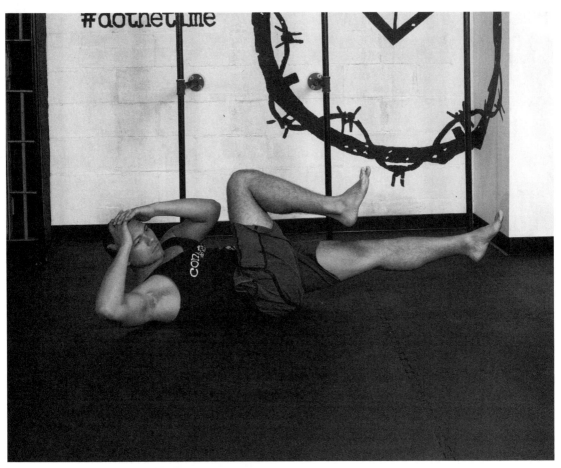

Supine bicycle.

Roll onto your back. Tuck your legs in at a 90-degree angle. Interlock your fingers in front of your forehead.

Kick one leg out. Bring opposite leg back.

Reach with opposite elbow so that it connects with the leg you bring back.

Repeat with opposite side.

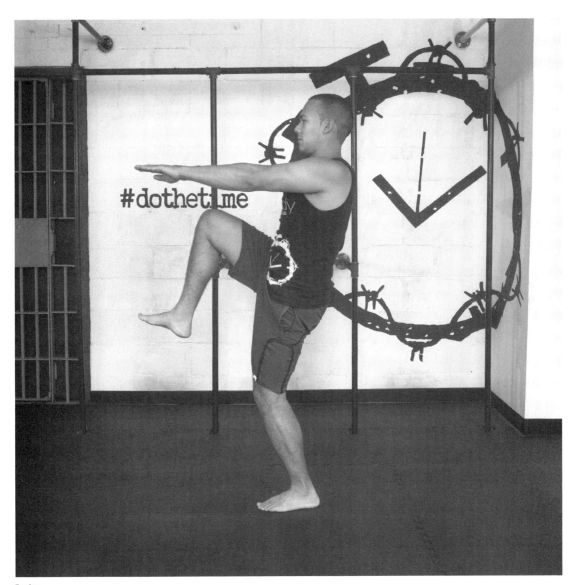

Engine.

Stand up. Put hands directly in front of you. Raise them up so that your arms are directly in front of you.

Bring one knee up to the same arm. Then bring that knee down, and repeat with opposite knee and opposite arm.

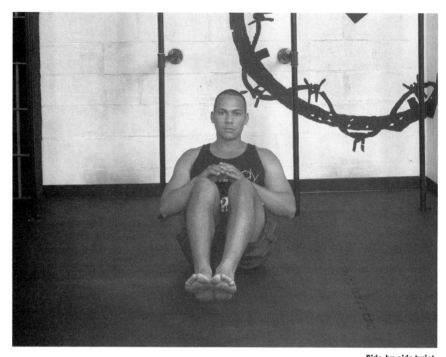

Side-by-side twist.
Sit on the ground. Bring your feet up about six inches.
Bring hands toward middle of your chest. Touch the ground from side to side.

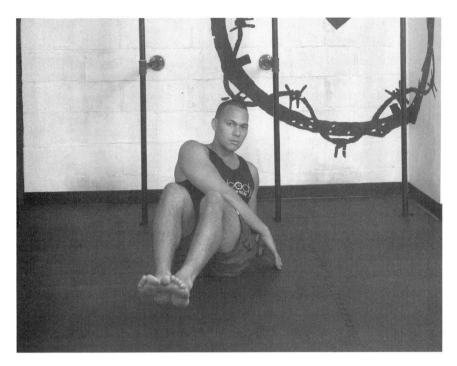

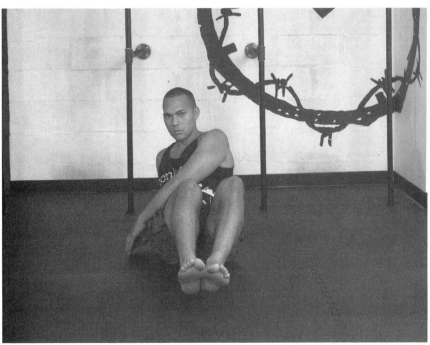

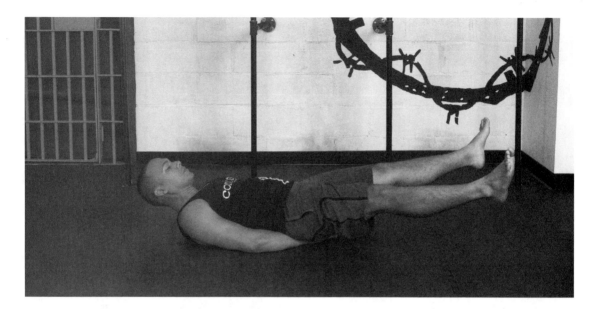

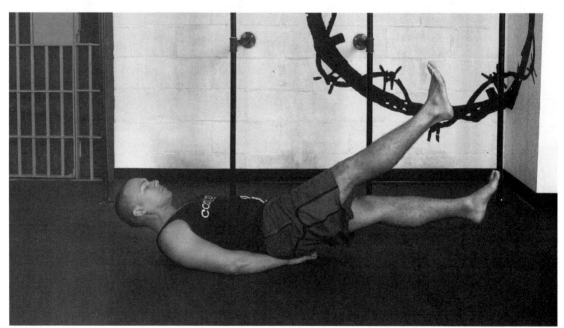

Flutter kick.
Lie flat on your back, hands under your butt. Feet six inches off the ground at starting position.
Bring one leg up and the other down—but without touching the ground—and then switch. Repeat.

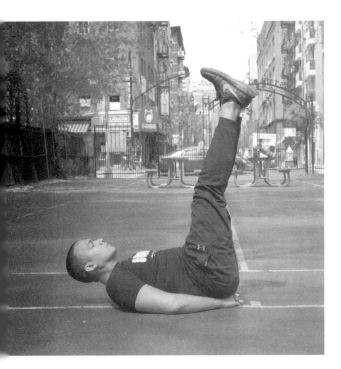

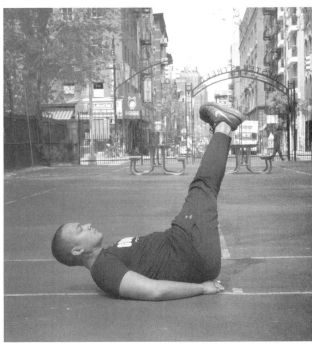

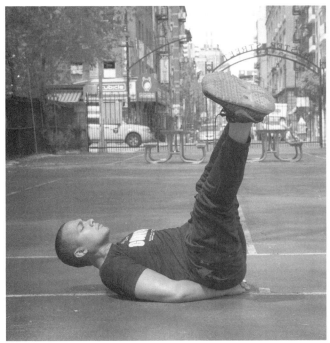

Windshield wiper.
Lie flat on your back, hands under your butt.
Legs straight up in the air. Then lower legs side to side,
barely touching the ground, then bring your legs up,
and go down to the other side. Repeat.
Make sure to keep both feet together.

Scissor kick up-and-down.
Lie flat on back, hands under butt,
feet six inches off the ground.
Spread legs.
Then close legs.
Then raise legs 45 degrees higher
than six inches.
Spread legs and close them. Bring
legs back down.
Spread legs and then close them.
Raise legs back up, and so on.

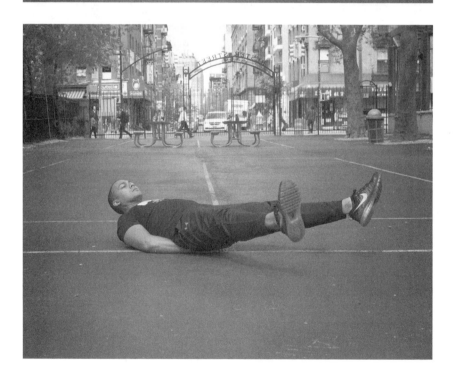

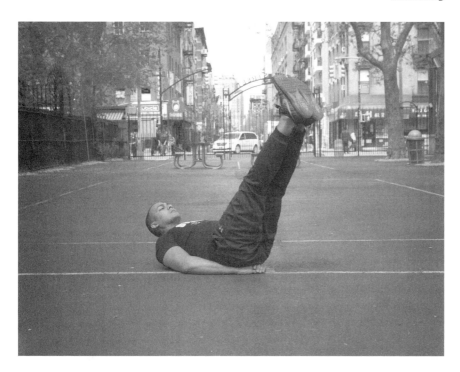

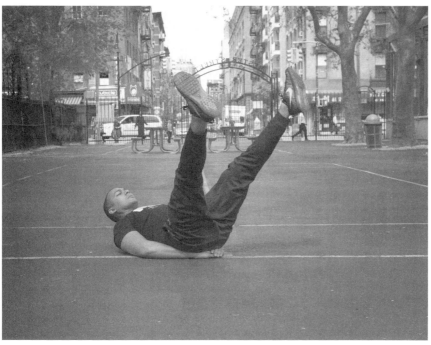

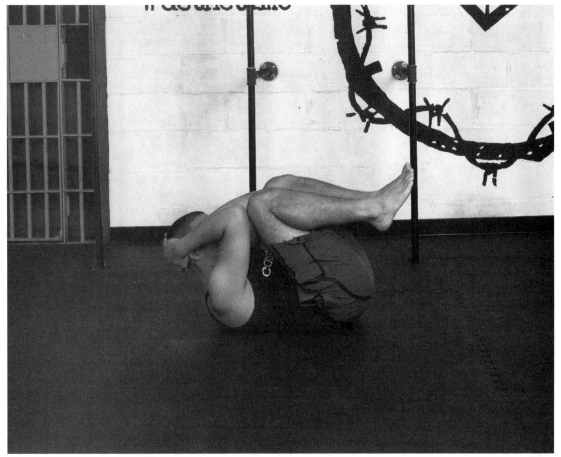

Crunch.

Lie flat on your back. Tuck in your legs. Keep your feet flat on the ground. Hold hands at temples. Keep them there as you crunch up. Bring your knees and elbows together.

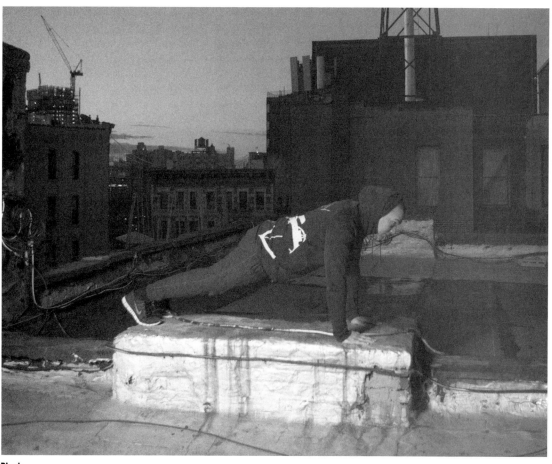

Plank.
Face the ground, holding yourself up like in the start of a push-up. Keep back flat. Hold.

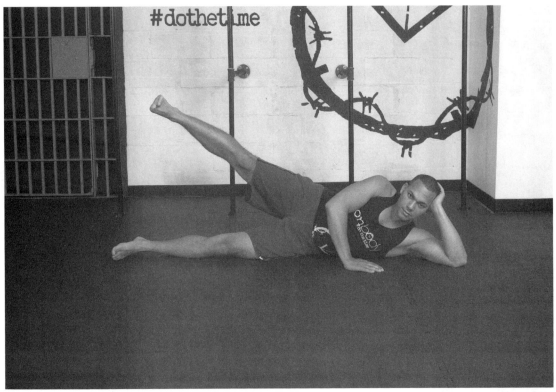

Side leg raise.
Lie down on your side.
Have your elbow and your arm
at a 90-degree angle.
Bring your top foot straight up toward the sky,
then bring it back down so your feet connect. Repeat.

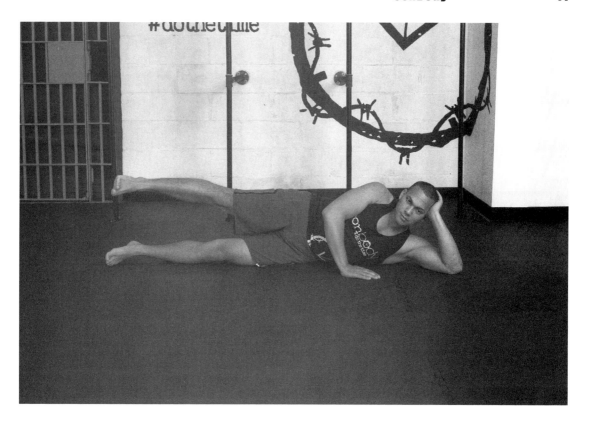

T-bone.

Sit. Place hands on ground beside your butt, directly below your shoulders. Lift your butt off the ground and hold yourself up with your hands, and kick your feet straight out in front of you so that your legs are fully extended. Then kick legs apart, similar to a scissor kick. Then bring legs back together, and then pull them back toward your body. Repeat.

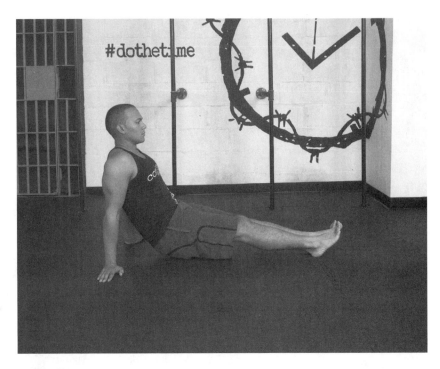

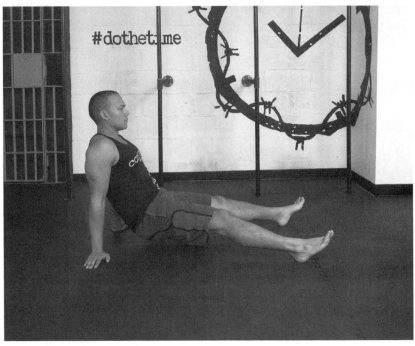

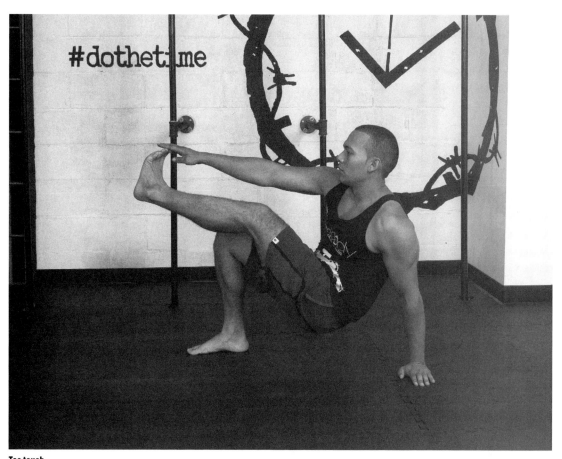

Toe touch.

Same starting position as a T-bone. Raise one foot off the ground and use opposite hand to touch toes.
Bring them back to the ground, then repeat with opposite side.

Back and forth.

Go down into push-up position, hands directly beneath shoulders, knees off the ground.

With a small jump, tuck your legs up underneath your stomach so that your feet land beneath you. With your hands on the ground behind you to hold you up, kick your feet straight out so they land with your legs fully extended, similar to the start of the T-bone. From there, pick up one of your hands and turn your body around, then place the hand back on the ground, so that you are then in the push-up position.

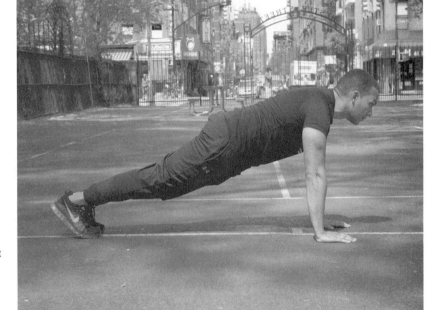

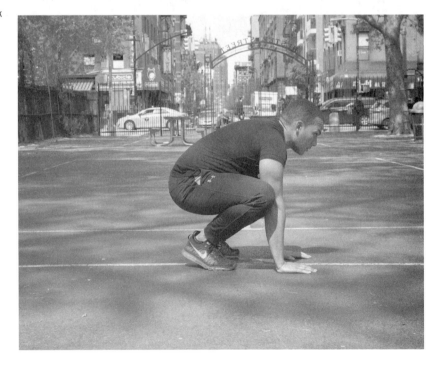

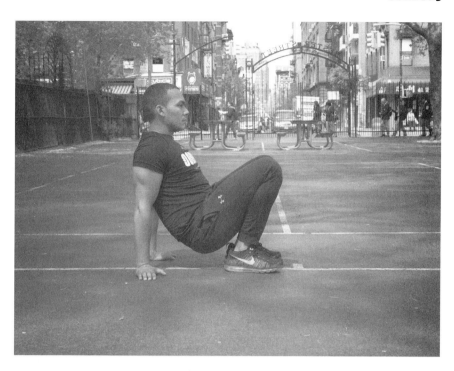

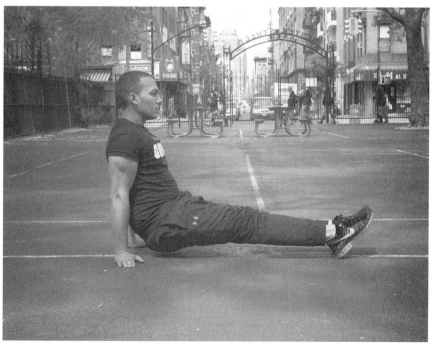

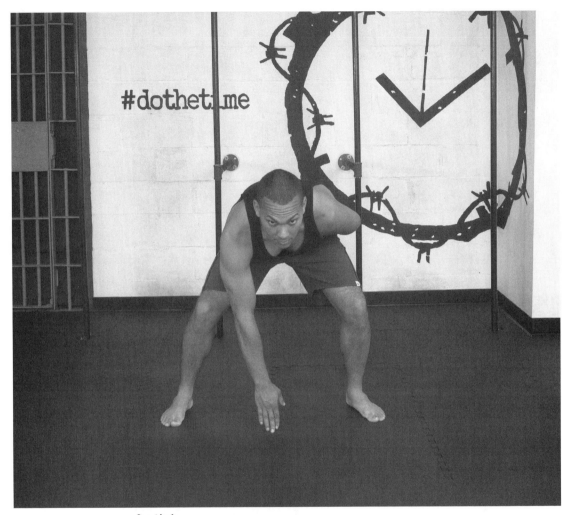

Squat jack.
Feet together, hands by your side, one hand directly over the center of your waist. Spread your legs and squat down. Touch the ground. Then close legs. Then spread them again and repeat, switching arms.

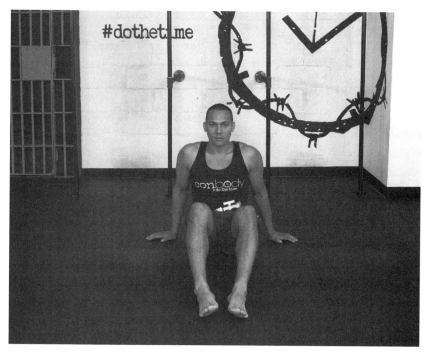

Up-and-down.
Sit on the ground, both hands behind your back. Then stand back up, putting the pressure on one arm. Repeat.
(Put same pressure on each arm, so if you go down on right hand 10 times, you also go down on left 10 times.)

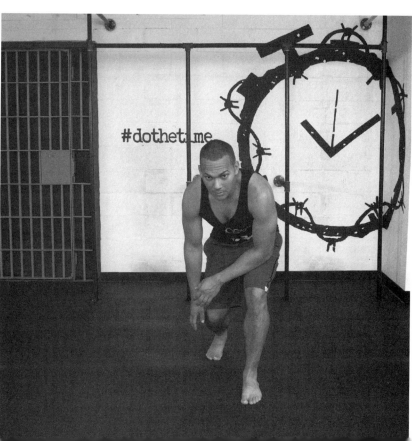

CARD GAME

I also started using the Card Game as a way to keep my work-outs fresh and different so that I didn't get bored, and so that my body didn't get too used to the same routine. That helped me burn weight and get back in shape faster.

Each card level means a certain number of reps:

▼ Jokers = 25

▼ Aces = 20

▼ Kings = 13

▼ Queens = 12

▼ Jacks = 11

▼ 10 down to 2 = 10

Each suit represents a certain exercise:

Lower Body

▼ Diamonds = Squat jacks

▼ Spades = Up-and-down

▼ Hearts = Squat thrust

▼ Clovers = 8-count lunge

▼ Jokers = Your choice

Upper Body

▼ **Various push-ups, your choice of diamond push-ups, wide push-ups, knuckle push-ups, fingertip push-ups, etcetera—and, of course, regular push-ups. For example:**

▼ Spades = Regular push-up

▼ Diamonds = Diamond push-up

▼ Hearts = Knuckle push-up

▼ Clovers = Wide push-up

▼ Jokers = Your choice

CARD GAME
PHOTOS

Pictures of the following lower body exercises can be found on earlier pages:

▼ Squat jack (page 82)

▼ Up-and-down (page 83)

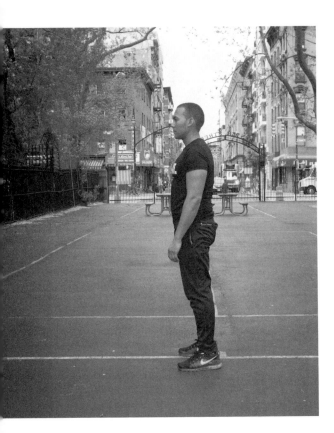
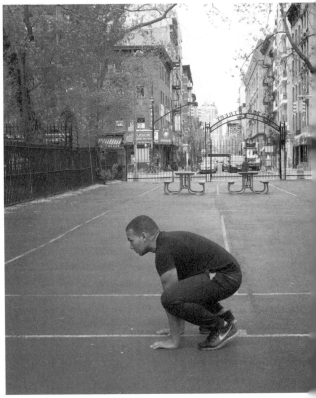

Squat thrust.
Stand up straight. Then squat down, putting your hands to the ground directly beneath you.
Thrust back into push-up position. Then thrust legs back into squatting position. Stand up.

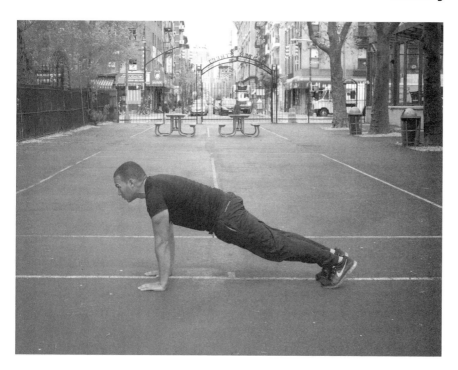

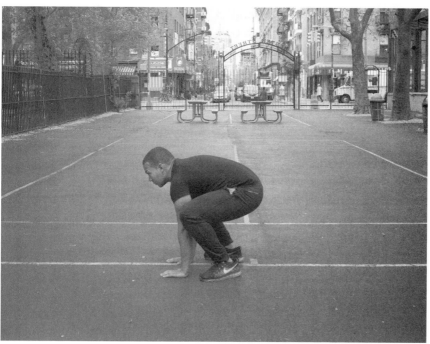

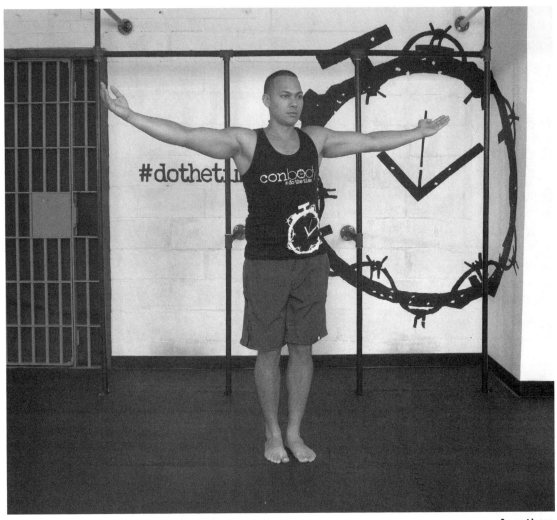

8-count lunge.
Put feet together. Hands by your side. Open up both arms, like a shoulder stretch position.
Extend one leg toward your right side, bringing your knee down to the ground.
Tuck both arms under your leg, so your elbows touch. Then stand back up to starting position.
Repeat on opposite side.

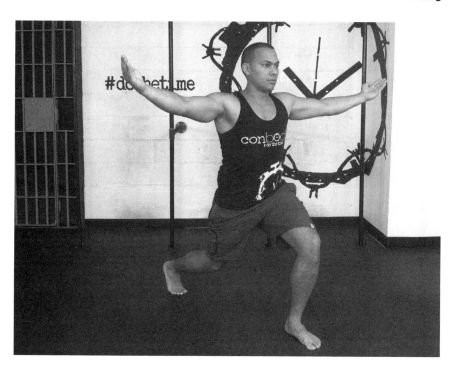

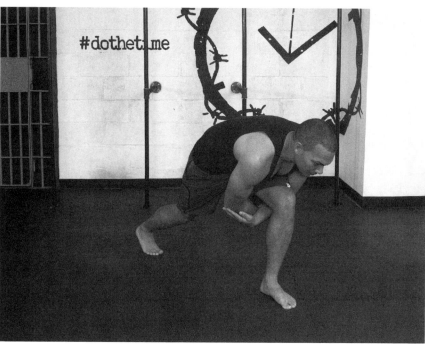

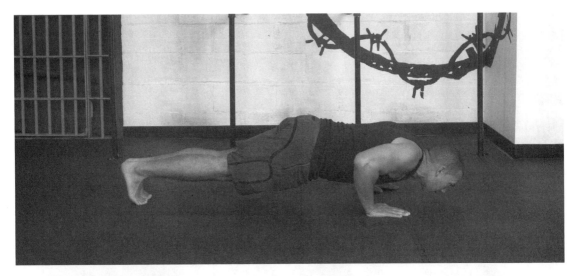

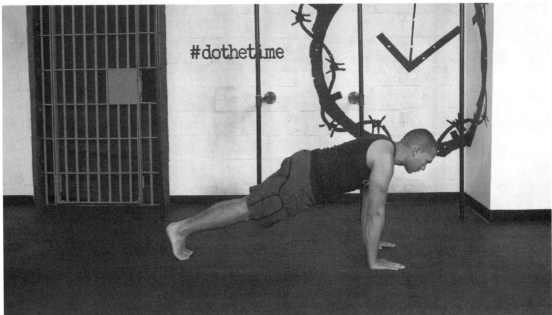

Regular push-up.
Lay down belly on the ground. Place your hands at your shoulders. Position your arms so that your elbows are at roughly a 90-degree angle and tucked against your side. Push up. Your entire body should leave the ground.
Keep your back flat. Keep your elbows tucked in to your sides instead of letting them spread out sideways. Go up and down, chest to the ground then back up.

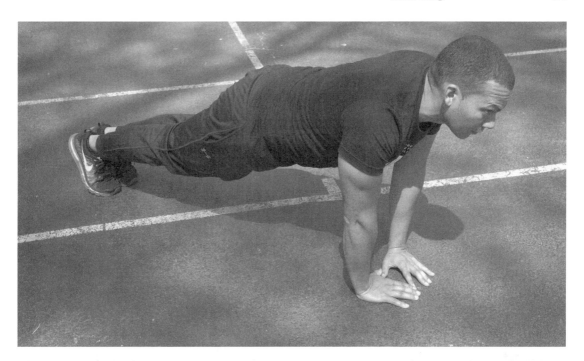

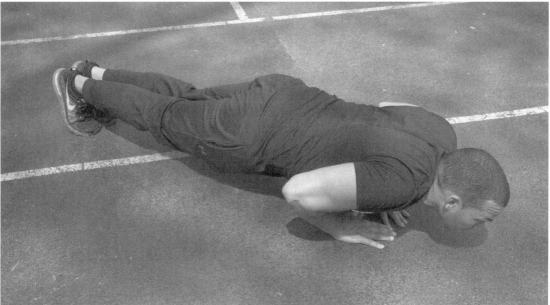

Diamond push-up.
Same as Regular, only bring your hands together beneath your chest and place them so that the thumbs and index fingers
touch, forming a diamond.

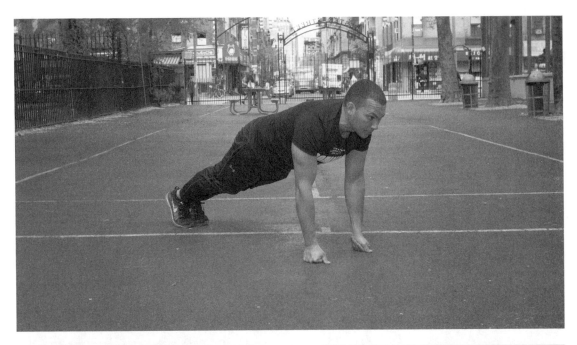

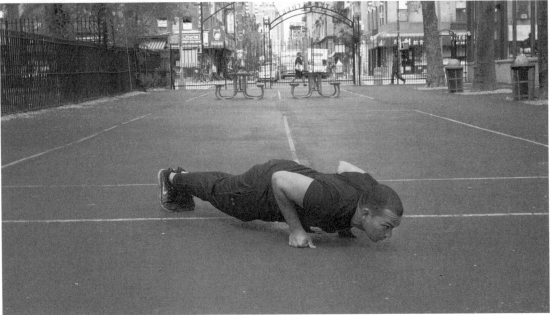

Knuckle push-up.
Same as Regular, only make a fist and do push-ups on flat knuckles instead of on your palms.

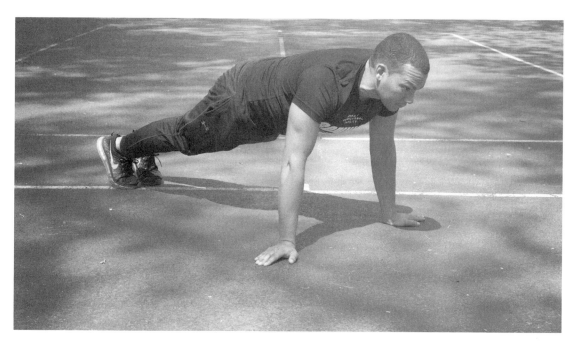

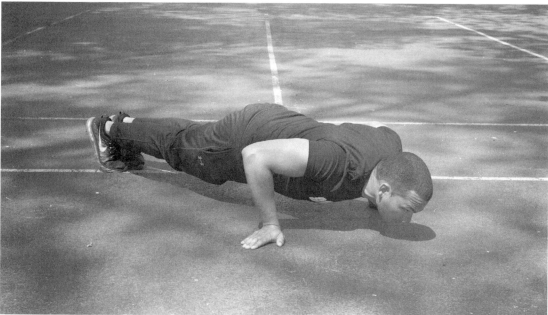

Wide push-up.
Same as Regular, only spread your hands a few hand widths beyond your shoulders, and turn your fingers so that they point to
the side instead of pointing forward.

4

MONTHS FOUR, FIVE, AND SIX

The Last Thirty Pounds

Losing forty pounds made me feel great. Healthier, lighter, more in control.

And some days, because of that, I felt like I was hitting a plateau, and some days, I felt like just coasting because I knew I was in better shape now.

But I wanted to find ways to keep pushing myself, to keep going.

||||||||

Around this time, I read in *Men's Health* that we burn something like 70 percent more body fat on an empty stomach, so I started making myself do a full ab workout before eating breakfast. Some days, I didn't eat until 11:00 a.m.

I tried to get in between 160–200 reps or more before I ate. Mostly I did the ab workouts that were listed in the "Core" section earlier, starting on page 62.

I would crank through 25–30 or more sets, five each of five different exercises.

I soon started to see some real definition in my core.

I also kept running. Some days, I'd run as many laps as I could during our two-hour blocks of time out in the yard (twice a day). Whenever we were out in the yard, I was working out all the time.

Then I started doing a game called "21 Down," where you do twenty-one push-ups, then rest by doing a plank hold while your partner does twenty-one push-ups—my partner at the time was my cell mate—and then you do twenty push-ups, then rest again holding a plank while your partner does his or her twenty push-ups, and so on, all the way down to one push-up.

Then you go all the way back up to twenty-one.

Come month five, I kept up the routine, and just kept making it more intense by however I could imagine. I even started using my bunk in my cell to do bench presses. I'd crawl underneath the bottom bunk and pump the whole thing up and down like a barbell.

Some days, I'd go through whole workouts in my cell with my mattress strapped to my back, like the crazy Marines had made us do during Shock. I'd run in place, do step-ups on the bunk, and do everything else I could possibly do carrying that extra weight.

In the yard, I started using light poles to run suicide-style sprints—similar to how basketball players use the free-throw line, half-court line, far free-throw line, and far baseline, running to one, touching it, running back to the baseline, touching it, and running to the next one and back, and so on.

And during the light pole sprints I started mixing in other exercises, too, as I rested between sets, such as:

▼ **Push-up walk**

▼ **Plank climbers crawl**

▼ **Bear crawl**

▼ **In and out**

▼ **Lunge walk**

▼ **Sideways crawl with toe touch**

▼ **Frog leap**

▼ **Bunny hop**

IIIIIIII

Around month five, I started using some of the prison weights maybe once a week.

Some days, when winter fell, I was the only guy out in the yard. Not just the only person working out—the only person out there, period. It gets really cold in upstate New York.

Guys walking by for programs or work stopped and stared. Some of them said I was crazy. When I jogged by the S-Block guys, they kept yelling at me, too, and even cussing me out.

I just kept going.

And within six months, I'd lost seventy pounds, the doctors told me I'd be just fine, and I could go out there and do forty pull-ups and look at the S-Block crew, and they didn't have anything they could say to me anymore.

TIER 3
SUPERMAX LEVEL WORKOUTS

Mix these in with Tiers 1 and 2.

Core

▼ 200+ reps doing 25+ sets of 5+ exercises from the "Core" section on pages 60–61. (Before breakfast if possible.)

Full Body

Superset each set with 1 set of suicide sprints (detailed below): 5 sets total if possible.

▼ Push-up walk

▼ Plank climbers crawl

▼ Bear crawl

▼ Lunge walk

▼ Sideways crawl with toe touch

▼ Frog leap

▼ Bunny hop

Suicide Sprints

▼ These can be done using just about anything as a marker. I used light poles. Basketball courts use the baseline, near foul line, half-court line, far foul line, and opposite baseline. Whatever you use, generally try to have your markers around 25, 50, 75, and 100 feet from the starting point.

From starting line, sprint to 25 feet, back to starting line, then back to 50, back to start, and so on up to 100, then back down to 25 before finishing.

21 Down

▼ Do 21 push-ups

▼ Rest while partner does 21 push-ups

▼ Repeat, decreasing by 1 push-up every set

▼ At 1 push-up, begin increasing by 1 push-up each set

▼ Finished after reaching 21 push-ups again

Push-up walk.
Squat. Do push-up.
Then thrust your legs into squatting position.
Then crawl out your hands all the way into next push-up position.
Then do another push-up.
Then jump into squatting position, and crawl out.

TIER 3
EXERCISE PHOTOS

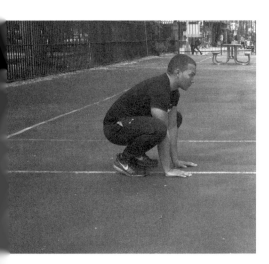 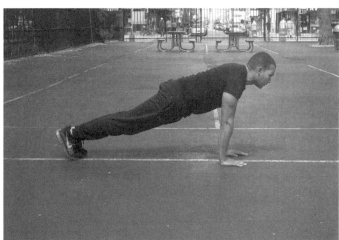

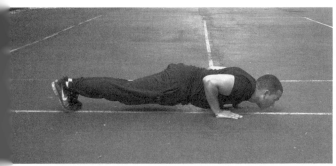 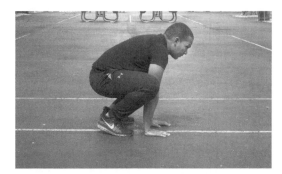

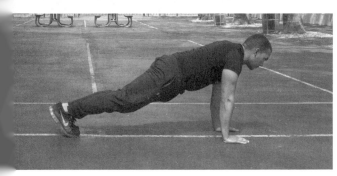 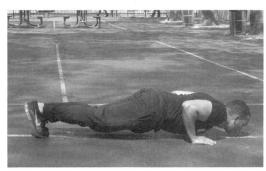

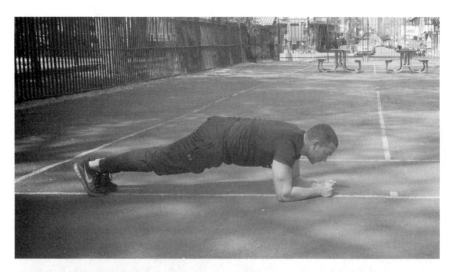

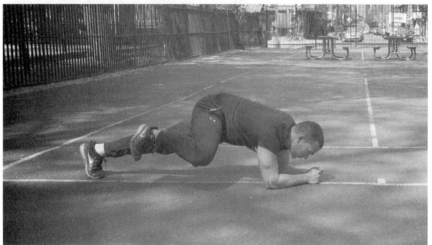

Plank climbers crawl.
Elbows down on the ground into a plank position.
Bring your knee toward your elbow on the same right
(i.e., right knee to right elbow).
Then go back to plank. Then left knee to left elbow.
Every time, take two steps with elbows, then do it again.

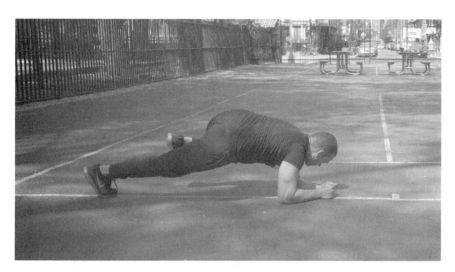

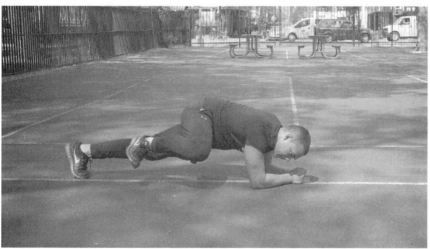

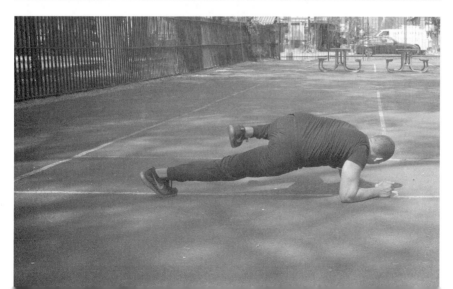

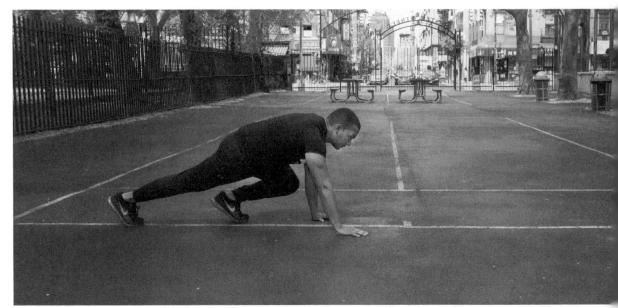

Bear Crawl.
From push-up position, crawl on toes and hands.
Bring one arm and its opposite leg forward
(i.e., left arm, right leg, or vice versa).
Move them back and forth as you crawl across the ground,
switching out and crawling without your knees, just your feet and hands.

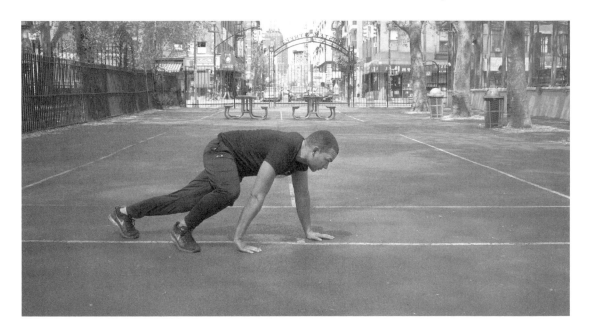

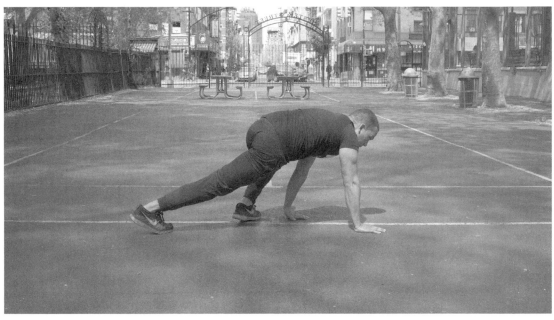

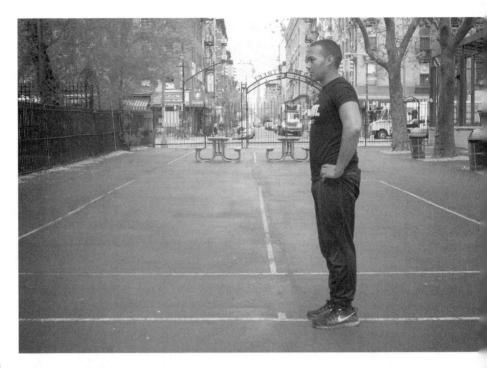

Lunge walk.
Standing, both feet together, hands on hips. Step forward so your lead knee is 90 degrees in front and your trailing knee is 90 degrees behind. Bring rear foot forward so your feet are side by side again. Step forward again using opposite foot of previous step. Repeat.

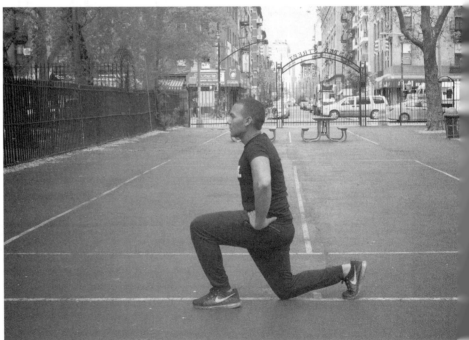

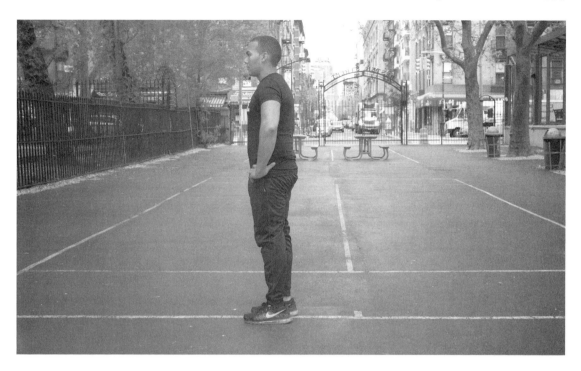

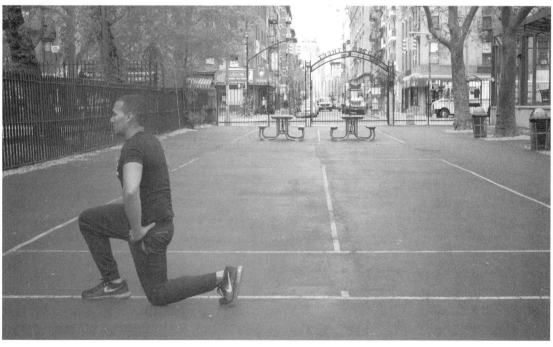

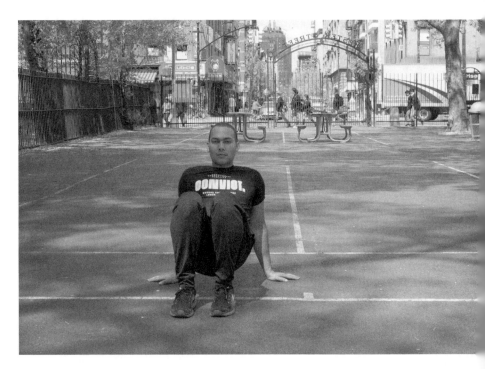

Sideways crawl with toe touch.
Sitting down, bring butt off the ground, with hands placed directly behind your back. Move sideways, same arm at the same time as the same leg (i.e., right leg moving forward with right arm). Stay on heels and hands, keeping your butt off the ground. With each step, also intermittently raise one foot off the ground and use opposite hand to touch its toes.

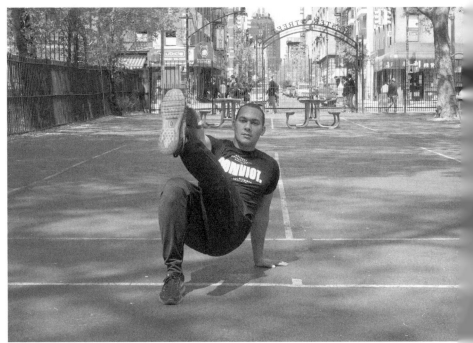

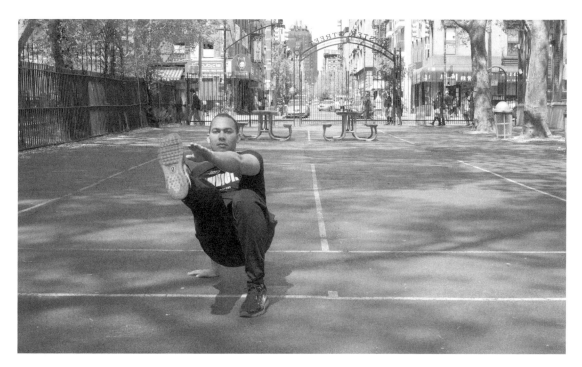

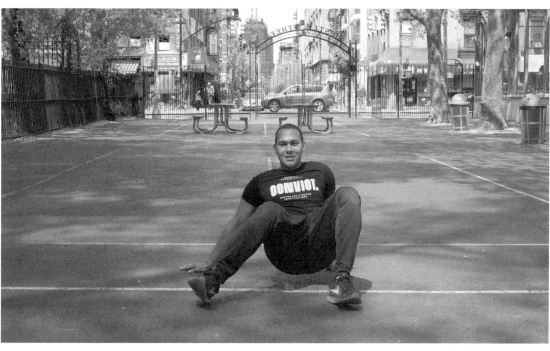

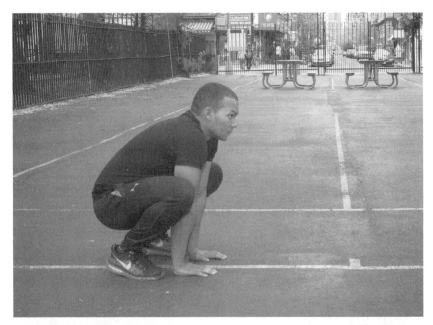

Frog leap.
From squatting position, lean onto
your toes. Place your hands directly
beneath you on the ground. Thrust
and jump forward. Land on your toes
and your hands.

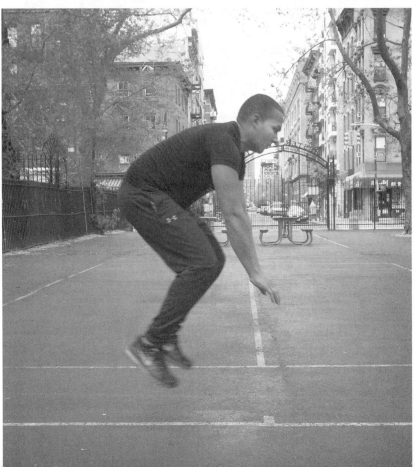

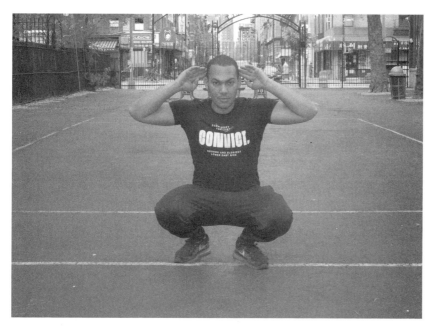

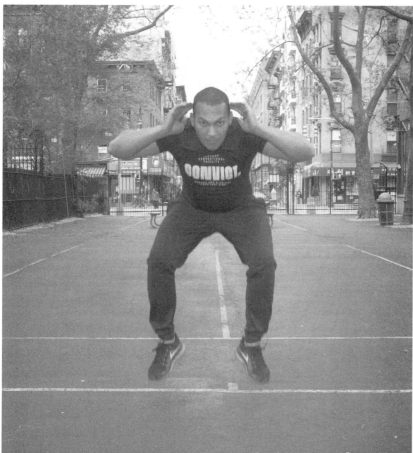

Bunny hop.
Squatting position, on your toes, with hands held up by the head for balance—then squat all the way down, so your butt is nearly on the ground. Hop forward using small hops.

21 DOWN
PUSH-UP GAME

Do 21 push-ups.

Rest while partner does 21 push-ups.

Do 20 push-ups.

Rest while partner does 20 push-ups.

Do 19 push-ups.

Rest while partner does 19 push-ups.

Do 18 push-ups.

Rest while partner does 18 push-ups.

Do 17 push-ups.

Rest while partner does 17 push-ups.

Do 16 push-ups.

Rest while partner does 16 push-ups.

Do 15 push-ups.

Rest while partner does 15 push-ups.

Do 14 push-ups.

Rest while partner does 14 push-ups

Do 13 push-ups

Rest while partner does 13 push-ups.

Do 12 push-ups.

Rest while partner does 12 push-ups.

Do 11 push-ups.

Rest while partner does 11 push-ups.

Do 10 push-ups.

Rest while partner does 10 push-ups.

Do 9 push-ups.

Rest while partner does 9 push-ups.

Do 8 push-ups.

Rest while partner does 8 push-ups.

Do 7 push-ups.

Rest while partner does 7 push-ups.

Do 6 push-ups.

Rest while partner does 6 push-ups.

Do 5 push-ups.

Rest while partner does 5 push-ups.

Do 4 push-ups.

Rest while partner does 4 push-ups.

Do 3 push-ups.

Rest while partner does 3 push-ups.

Do 2 push-ups.

Rest while partner does 2 push-ups.

Do 1 push-up.

Rest while partner does 1 push-up.

Do 2 push-ups.

Rest while partner does 2 push-ups.

Do 3 push-ups.

Rest while partner does 3 push-ups.

Do 4 push-ups.

Rest while partner does 4 push-ups.

Do 5 push-ups.

Rest while partner does 5 push-ups.

Do 6 push-ups.

Rest while partner does 6 push-ups.

Do 7 push-ups.

Rest while partner does 7 push-ups.

Do 8 push-ups.

Rest while partner does 8 push-ups.

Do 9 push-ups.

Rest while partner does 9 push-ups.

Do 10 push-ups.

Rest while partner does 10 push-ups.

Do 11 push-ups.

Rest while partner does 11 push-ups.

Do 12 push-ups.

Rest while partner does 12 push-ups.

Do 13 push-ups.

Rest while partner does 13 push-ups.

Do 14 push-ups.

Rest while partner does 14 push-ups.

Do 15 push-ups.

Rest while partner does 15 push-ups.

Do 16 push-ups.

Rest while partner does 16 push-ups.

Do 17 push-ups.

Rest while partner does 17 push-ups.

Do 18 push-ups.

Rest while partner does 18 push-ups.

Do 19 push-ups.

Rest while partner does 19 push-ups.

Do 20 push-ups.

Rest while partner does 20 push-ups.

Do 21 push-ups.

Rest while partner does 21 push-ups.

5

KEEPING IT OFF

So by the end of 2009, I was set, healthy, and ready to go.

But keeping the weight off and not resorting to old, bad habits is always tough. I would get so bored in there. I would get so tired of trying to eat healthy.

You think healthy food tastes bad compared to junk food on the outside? Try to imagine how bad it tastes when the unhealthy food in prison already tastes terrible.

I was constantly tempted to start making Prison Burritos again.

And to be clear, I wasn't exactly an angel all the time. I was still getting weed from COs or from what buddies smuggled in. I was still dealing, too—and I'd started a low-key prison hooch business.

But I knew I had to stay in shape, because I wanted to start Shock again as soon as they'd let me—but I knew I had no chance of making it through if I got anywhere close to being as fat and unhealthy as I had been.

What motivated me as much as anything, though, weren't my

own goals and hopes, but also helping other people. I think one of the most important keys to staying healthy, for all of us, is this: Ultimately, it has to be not only about ourselves, but also about making ourselves better so that we are better for people that we love, and who love us.

For me, there were three things that kept me going.

IIIIIIIII

First, Lil C.

The worst part of prison was having to watch him grow up from across a table and only seeing him every so often.

His mom would bring him to visit and we'd spend as much time as we could together. Sometimes the guards would have to force me to leave the visitation area because it broke my heart to leave him.

And then he would be crying and when he started talking it got even worse because he could ask me to stay.

Sometimes he would scream and run after me until the guards carried *him* out. And even then he would try to beat them up with his little fists.

I wanted to take him to Yankees games and tuck him in at night and tell him stories to help him fall asleep.

IIIIIIIII

The second thing that kept me going was training other guys. If Lil C gave me a grand sense of purpose in the big-picture sense, then the guys on the inside trying to get and stay in shape with me were my day-to-day inspiration.

There'd be a whole group of us, a half dozen or more, going through the Card Game and running sprints and doing pull-ups, all of us helping each other, and running ten laps at a time around the track, pushing each other.

I remember one guy in particular named Almonte. He was Dominican like me and came in weighing like three hundred pounds. And he was shorter than me, so he was really round. We got to be friends in 2012 and eventually he saw me working out and started talking about wanting to lose weight, too, but saying how impossible it was. So I told him my story and how I'd lost so much weight.

He didn't believe me at first, but then I pulled out my old prison ID and showed him. And he still didn't believe me. But then he did, and we started working out together.

All in all, I helped about twenty guys lose about a thousand pounds total.

And we didn't even always work out hard-core. Some days, we just played basketball and football.

And soccer.

Mannn, I'd missed it. As I'd lost weight, I'd starting feeling that little kid in me come back alive again. That felt a little strange, too, because I realized that little kid was way farther gone than I could've imagined.

But without even realizing it, I was planning to lock that little kid in me away again as soon as I got out.

IIIIIIIII

The third thing that kept me going was knowing that when I got out, I had learned enough to avoid getting caught again.

After all, I'd been doing masterful work inside beyond working out. Even as I was getting in shape again, I was also running a successful inmate weed and hooch business.

I'd made a mistake to get caught and land back in here: I trusted the wrong guy, who led the feds right to me. I believed I could out-smart them moving forward. So when I got out, I was going to return to my broken empire and rebuild.

Soon as I was eligible, I jumped into Shock again.

It did not go well.

6

SHOCK

Watching Lil C leave crying after his visits with me was the worst part of prison, but there's a difference between worst and hardest.

The *hardest* part of prison was tolerating most of the guards.

If any of us inmates moved wrong, spoke wrong, or otherwise did something the guards deemed wrong, we'd get cracked and then face two choices: fight back or fight down our survival instincts and take the beating. If we retaliated, though, then they'd sound the alarm and other guards would come and the beating would get worse.

We didn't even have to *actually* retaliate—we just had to *appear* as though we could *maybe* be *thinking* about it, and they'd sound the alarm.

And with the alarm would also come the inevitable sentence in solitary confinement.

In August 2012, I was only a few weeks away from finishing the Shock program again, and Lil C had just come for a visit. He didn't want to leave when our time was up, and his mom had to carry him away crying. I called after him, saying I was almost done, little buddy, and I'd be home soon for good.

Then I went to the medical unit for what I thought would be a routine dental exam, but instead an officer handed me a pee cup for a surprise drug test. It was a dirty trick, but I wasn't worried because I stopped sneaking weed once I started Shock again.

But it took me a minute to pee, especially with this guard standing right over my shoulder staring at my junk, and he was in a bad mood and snapped at me, "Don't waste my fucking time."

Then—I don't even know what happened next. Maybe I said something he didn't like, or took the wrong way, but I don't know what I did to set him off. All I know is, he said, "Don't fuck with me. I'm not having a good day." Then I was on the ground and my glasses had flown off somewhere, and my head was ringing. The back of my head hurt and I could feel it swelling.

I turned around, dizzy and confused, and saw the officer shaking out his fist like he'd just punched someone.

He reared up again and barked at me, "You turning around on me?! You gonna do something?!"

I told him no, and I lowered my head and spread my hands like I was bowing or something.

I asked him to please stop, and said I didn't want any problems. I was ready to go home and didn't want this idiot messing that up for me.

It didn't matter.

He flipped a switch on his radio, and there went the alarm.

A bunch more officers poured into the bathroom and beat me up.

Then they threw me in solitary.

||||||||||

That meant I was kicked out of Shock.

Worse, the officer wrote me up for refusing a drug test and fighting an officer.

That's a Tier 3 ticket, the worst level.

I've known guys who spent a whole year in solitary for a Tier 3 ticket.

7

ADDICTION

As much as it is about anything else, this book is about addiction.

And it's about the type of people that we've become that allow us to become unhealthy, and about the type of people we need to become before we can actually be what we want to be.

The reality is that none of us become fat and out of shape and deathly unhealthy by choice, and most of us know we're headed down that deadly path—but we also feel powerless to stop it. Somehow, we have gotten locked into patterns of behavior and eating and motionlessness that we feel powerless to break out of.

We have become addicted.

And in this addiction, we become something completely different from what we thought we were, from what we saw for ourselves—so far from where we thought we were going.

Even if we somehow find the strength to take the steps we need to take to break away from all of that, somewhere along the way, as you lose the weight you want to lose and transform into the person you hoped you could actually be—*boom*—things will happen that will push you off track and threaten to wreck you all over again.

You will either return to old habits—by giving in to old addictions—or lean forward into your new ones. You will go forward, or you will go backward. And if you go backward, that's like starting to die all over again.

There are a lot of different ways that we can be imprisoned—and not only by other people, but by ourselves.

These are hard lessons to learn, but as much as any exercise, they are crucial lessons about what it also takes to break free and become who you are trying to be. I hope that—somehow—my simply putting those words on this page helps you.

I also didn't realize that my actions were putting others in prison, too—a different sort of prison, but a prison nonetheless. I'm hardheaded like that, and back then, as if you couldn't tell by now, I hated admitting I was wrong about anything. This was my most valuable lesson, and it was the hardest one for me to learn, because learning this lesson happened just a few short weeks before I should have been released. Instead, I got thrown into solitary.

||||||||

All I had in solitary was paper and a pen and a Bible. I wrote my family a ten-page letter telling them what happened and that I wouldn't be home and telling Lil C that I loved him. I missed him so much.

But I didn't have a stamp so I couldn't even give it to the guard to put in the mail.

After five days in solitary, I got a letter from my sister. She wrote about Psalm 91. "Please go read it," she said. "Read it and pray."

I tossed the letter aside and ignored it.

Of course, being in solitary, I soon got bored, so I then opened the Bible and turned to Psalm 91.

A stamp fell out.

I got chills.

Then I read.

And then more chills.

|||||||||

*Whoever dwells in the shelter of the Most High will
rest in the shadow of the Almighty. I will say of the Lord,
"He is my refuge and my fortress, my God, in whom I trust."
Surely he will save you.*

|||||||||

I kept reading for days. All of Psalms and Proverbs, then half
the New Testament.

I read 1 Timothy 6:10: *The love of money is the root of all kinds of
evil.*

Then I remembered things I'd learned about addiction.

|||||||||

Psychology classes and books taught me that there's a cluster of
cells in our brains—called the "nucleus accumbens"—which gets
dosed with the neurotransmitter "dopamine" when we do something fun, like have sex or eat a donut.

Dopamine is known as "the pleasure chemical," which is what
makes you feel so good.

Thing is, we're designed to feel those kinds of highs, and maybe
even to experience this kind of addiction. The key is to experience it with the right things, with healthy things. Because what
is addiction if not a commitment to something that causes you to
become numb and blind to other things that would take you away
from it?

Love is an addiction to another person. That's why breakups

suck so bad. That's why—God forbid—if my son died I would feel like dying, too.

And when I am with him and he is happy, I feel as high as I've ever felt after taking any drug.

This might be oversimplifying things a bit, but the good things we crave in life do cause the same sort of behavior in the brain as the bad things we can get addicted to. The chemicals in our brains that make us feel high are all already there—it's just a matter of what we do to release them, and knowing when the things we do to release them are helping or hurting us.

Drugs trigger the same response, especially crack and cocaine, and they trigger it with insane intensity, flooding the nucleus accumbens. That's getting high.

And get high like that all the time, you'll wear out the nerve cells until the brain has to shut things down, cutting off the dopamine flow from everything. Life goes gray and the world feels dead, and nothing can resurrect you until you get a hit of the drug again.

And some people are way more sensitive, and become addicted to things much more easily. Maybe not even to drugs, but any number of vices.

Gambling. Violence. Sex.

Greasy food. Soda. Chocolate.

All of these trigger those same feel-good drugs already waiting in your brain to be deployed so they can go swimming around in there, making you feel high.

These are the types of people who become hard-core addicts; the same ones who became my best customers.

The hard-core addict ends up overusing the dopamine receptors until the nerves die.

Then they need more and more to breach the brain's dopamine dams until they need so much their body can't handle it, and then they die.

|||||||||

It was there, while I was in solitary—reading that Bible verse, remembering what I learned in psychology class—that I first took an honest look at what I had been doing. I realized two things.

One: Same as I know of addicts robbing and beating people, hurting people, to get money so they could get their drug, I was, in my own way, robbing and hurting the addicts I sold my drugs to. I wasn't treating them like people, but like customers, knowing their weakness and preying upon it, like a vulture, just so they would give me money so I would give them drugs that would make them feel free again—when in reality, I wasn't selling them freedom, I was selling them a lie, and only locking them away more.

I was hurting people for no reason other than making money.

Two: I was doing what I was doing because I was an addict, too.

My vice wasn't crack or some other drug.

My vice was money.

My brain had hijacked me.

I missed playing soccer and baseball. I missed being active and making those diving plays.

But I loved making money more.

The more I made and the more I learned how to make it, the more I wanted to make.

I'd thought I was living life just how I wanted.

After all, we had partied as hard as we worked. The Jordans. The Cadillac. The spontaneous trips to the Caribbean. The fight club. The f-ing Central Park horse and buggy and feeding the animal an apple pie. We were a crew better than rock stars and I was their boss. Coss the *Motherfucking* Boss.

But now I can't help but wonder: *Were we really having fun?*

Was there real joy in any of that?

Or did something in us know all along that what we were doing to make our money was wrong? Did something in us know that to prey upon the weaknesses of others, just to bleed them of money, and keep them under our control, so that they would only keep giving us more, until they had given all that they could, was wrong?

And were we really partying just because we felt like it and we could?

Or did we *need* the party, like another kind of drug, another addiction, to numb that knowing part of ourselves?

Did we need it to block our heart—to keep ourselves distracted so we didn't think, because if we could think, then we would see what we were doing?

Maybe.

Because the truth was, I was ruining lives. I had ruined my life. I was ruining my son's life.

For the dollar.

I felt flooded by waves of shame and sorrow and regret.

I couldn't believe how selfish I had been.

I wanted to break out of that cell and that prison and run home so that I could hug everyone.

My friends. My brother. My sisters. My parents. Everyone in my neighborhood. My addicted customers.

My son.

I wanted to hug them and tell them what I found myself telling God right then in that solitary cell.

I'm sorry.

I repent.

I'll make this right.

8

RECOVERY

Not knowing how long I'd be in solitary and trying to not go crazy in there, I started working out all the time, even more than before.

I had to get creative to keep my workouts fresh (not to mention to keep my mind from going numb). I invented exercise moves that, if they do exist somewhere, I'd never heard of before: T-bones, up-and-downs, and so on. They are included in the one-month ConBody boot camp section starting on page 131.

Maybe most importantly, I turned my addictive brain toward something productive.

||||||||

I still wanted to make money when I got out. I still wanted to be rich. But I wanted to get rich—unbelievable as this thought was to me at the time—*the right way.*

I wanted to do it in a way that, even if I *didn't* end up making much, it still allowed me to give something back to the world for what I'd done—starting with my neighborhood.

So I decided to start a fitness company when I got out.

I spent hours a day inventing various exercise regimens and writing them out on countless pieces of paper, thinking up all the best combinations.

||||||||

They let me out of solitary after thirty days.

When I got out, I was allowed back into Shock. I jumped right in, even though I had to start over again. I wasn't staying in prison any longer than I had to.

As I went through Shock for the third time, I couldn't help but talk about my new plans with the guys.

They told me, "You're fucking crazy" and that it was never going to work.

They knew the cold, harsh truth about the outside; the same truth I knew, which, in part, drove me to keep dealing after my first time in prison.

The world is different for felons, especially felons of color. It's not a world we realistically expect to thrive in. We know better than to get our hopes up. It's a world that we only try to survive.

I didn't accept that.

So I argued.

I told them to just watch me.

I told them that I started with an ounce of weed for a hundred bucks when I was a kid and I built that into a multimillion-dollar organization.

I told them I knew how to bust my ass.

I told them I knew how to make shit happen.

I finished Shock in March 2013 and went home. I was twenty-seven years old and starting completely over. And so my true test began.

||||||||

When you decide to move forward, you will still face setbacks and obstacles. You have to just keep going.

Maybe—and I hope this is true for you—it is as simple as to keep working out.

However, for many, as it was for me, it may also mean rebuilding your entire life. I just want you to know that you can actually do it. If I could, then you definitely can.

The good news is that those brain drugs can also be deployed by things like working out and helping people. I knew that it would take a while to break those old habits and make new ones, but when our brain learns the new healthy ways to get the same drugs and feel the same pleasure, then, in a sense, it gets addicted to those, too.

I knew I just had to do the time.

||||||||||

When I got out and went back home, my old crew didn't even recognize me at first. Funny how sometimes outgrowing a life means becoming less of something, not more of another thing.

Soon as I got home, the temptation to jump back into my old life clawed at me from the start. I'd learned how to better keep myself from getting caught again. How I could make that good money again; become a kingpin again; live life big again.

And it wasn't just the money and the good life that tempted me: It was just wanting to have my own life, a decent life.

I still had the connections.

I could have done it easily.

Plus, I had no money left.

And finding a job right away was impossible.

Nobody hires ex-cons (even if you promise potential employers that you wouldn't sell drugs at your new job with them).

I also had no clothes because all my old, nice clothes were way too big for me now.

I had to borrow money from my parents to buy old secondhand clothes again, like when I was a kid.

I couldn't even live with my son and then-girlfriend because her apartment was in the Bronx, in subsidized housing—I wasn't allowed to live in subsidized housing while on parole.

So I had to move back in with my parents, back in my old Lower East Side neighborhood. Lots of other guys were still around, asking me to start selling again.

But I didn't. I knew myself and my addictions. I'd renounced my old religion. I didn't want to go knee-deep in the crack game again.

Soon as I got home I started working out again.

I wanted to stay addicted to that.

||||||||

I got up every day at 5:30 a.m. and went for runs, and then went back to Roosevelt, the same park I used to use as home base for dealing, to work out there.

I followed the same workout routine that I created in prison—I wanted to stay committed to what had set me free so that I could stay free.

I started getting my mom up with me so that she could work out, too. She told a friend, and then her friend started working out with us. Maybe it's obvious, but no, I did not charge my mom. I didn't get paid for working out with anybody until some time after my boy Pilo got out of prison.

When he got out, he wanted to stay addicted to the clean life, too. He wanted to become a barber. So he started working out with me to stay focused.

We went back to Roosevelt once again, our old stomping grounds, first for soccer, then for dealing, and now for working out.

The park had no pull-up bar, so we made one out of an old pipe that we would slide through the links on the corner of a fence. Between that and some of the other crazy stuff we were doing, random people on the street started asking questions about our workouts, and I started training them, too.

Before long we had a whole group working out in the park together. Some of my old friends from the neighborhood, I trained for free—and as more and more strangers started asking questions, too, ConBody was born.

IIIIIIII

Part of my parole requirements were to connect with some nonprofits that would teach me how to apply for "real" jobs. I started at a Goodwill in Brooklyn as an unpaid intern for a few months until I convinced them to hire me full-time—and then, lo and behold, Coss the *Motherfucking* Boss had himself a nine-to-five.

Never thought I'd be so happy to have such a normal job.

Meanwhile, I built ConBody by getting up at 5:00 a.m. and hiking several blocks over to a studio space I rented, teaching classes for a couple of hours, then going to work, then returning to the studio that night to teach classes for a few more hours. (Some days, I held the classes at Roosevelt.)

Along the way, I also hooked up with Defy Ventures, a nonprofit that helps ex-cons like me channel their entrepreneurial skills in a legal way. And they have one of the best perspectives on ex-cons that I've ever come across. Their founder, Catherine Hoke, always says, "If you weren't any good at selling crack on the street corner, we probably don't want you." That line usually makes people laugh, but she's only half joking, because she knows that successful drug dealers and gang leaders have a lot of the same gifts as great businessmen and women.

At the end of their training, they hold a *Shark Tank*–style competition where we pitched our business concepts to grant givers. I won, which banked me $10,000. I used the money to make a website, to produce some swag, and to get my business in order.

Eventually I started renting ballet studios to train people there, too. I had to change up the routines because some of them were too hard for beginners.

About a year after I got out, I got my own place, a little apartment on Eldridge, just a couple of blocks from Roosevelt and maybe three blocks from my mom's place. Through Defy Ventures I hooked up with another *Shark Tank*–style competition led by real estate queen and "Shark" Barbara Corcoran—and I won that, too. And along the way, as I raised money with other private investors, I scored about $100,000 in early investments.

That felt as good to me as any deal I'd made dealing drugs. Frankly, everything felt almost exactly the same—I was just selling a different product now. (And I didn't have to worry about undercover cops arresting me, which was also nice.)

Since then, I've opened my own studio on the Lower East Side, still in the same hood where I once became a drug kingpin. Some people think it's risky, that I might fall back into old habits, but I like being right there, staring my old demons down, watching them fall behind like fat guys in a footrace. That's the thing about our demons: They're not that scary once we show them we can beat them.

I spoke everywhere, took every interview, watched as feature stories on popular websites and TV stations went viral. Even though it was what I was working for, it was still so surreal.

Soon there will be more ConBody studios. I have trained thousands of students and ConBody now trains some two hundred students a day and brings in around $500,000 a year.

Same as I addictively pursued the dollar selling blow on street corners, I addictively pursued clients and publicity and ConBody believers.

I built the business the same way, too, hitting the streets every chance I got, just like in my drug kingpin days. Only now, instead of slinging crack, I was selling a prison boot camp that came with a healthy side of hope and inspiration.

Extra! Extra! We got fitness!

IIIIIIIII

So that's how working out changed my life, and even saved it, not just because I lost weight, but because it gave me a life beyond prison.

I just had to do the time.

CONBODY BOOT CAMP
ONE-MONTH STARTER PLAN

Here is a basic and intensive ConBody starter boot camp.

You can customize however you want, using these exercises and/or others from throughout the book. (And remember that when you count these out, count military style: "One-two-three-ONE. One-two-three-TWO. One-two-three-THREE...")

Whatever exercises you do, the most important thing will always be the following: Just do the time.

Repeat every week for four weeks.

Manic Monday (30 minutes)

Do all exercises listed below without stopping.

▼ Twisted jumping jacks: 200 (as many as possible without stopping, then keep going)

▼ Calf raises with finger flicks: 100 (without stopping)

▼ Calf stretch toe pulls (standing): 10-count on each toe

▼ Up-and-downs: 20

▼ Groin stretches/wide hamstring stretches (standing): 10-count per side

▼ Stationary running: 200-count, while moving arms and legs

▼ Push-up claps: 30 *(if claps are too difficult, do regular push-ups)*

▼ Planks: 30-count

▼ **Push-up plank: hold the planks for a 30-count**

▼ **Lay-up-and-downs: 60-count, up and down**

30-second break.

Repeat.

MANIC MONDAY
PHOTOS

Pictures of the following Manic Monday exercises have already appeared:

- **Calf raise (page 36). To add "finger flicks," simply extend your arms out to your sides with a closed fist. Every time your heels go up, open your hands and fully extend your fingers. Close when your heels go down, then repeat.**

- **Calf stretch toe pull (page 21)**

- **Up-and-down (page 83)**

- **Groin stretch/wide hamstring stretch (page 27)**

- **Plank (page 75)**

- **Push-up plank: do push-up (page 41), then hold plank position for 30 seconds**

- **Lay-up-and-down (page 65)**

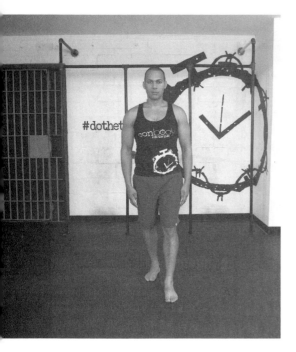

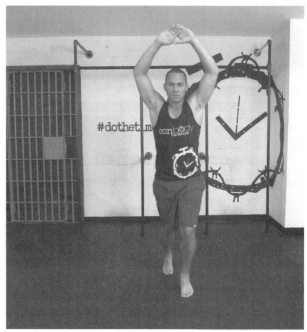

Twisted jumping jack.
One foot forward, one foot back, hands by your side.
Jump, bringing hands up so they connect over your head, and
switching legs so they go backward and forward,
landing in the opposite place from where they started.
As you land, bring your hands back down to your sides. Repeat.

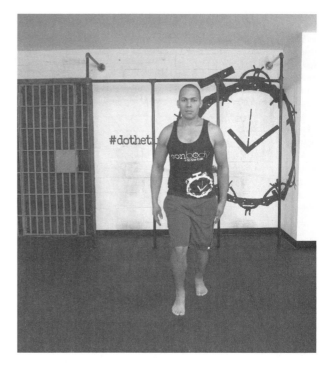

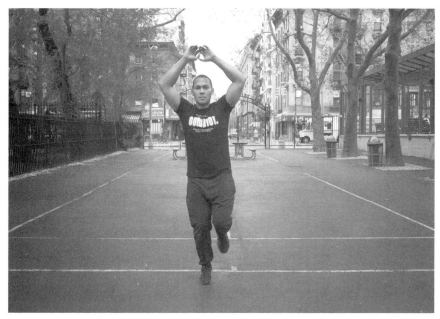

Stationary running.
Stand still in one spot. Move feet as though running, but do not actually go forward or backward. Bring heels and toes fully off the ground.

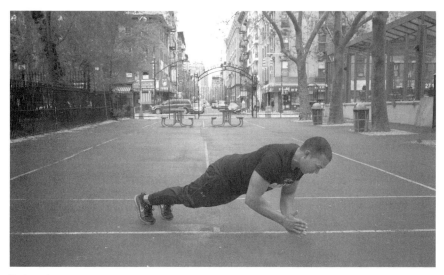

Push-up clap.
Push-up position. In the starting position—chest down, arms 90-degree angle—thrust body upward and bring your hands together so they clap. Then land in push-up position.

Tough-Love Tuesday (30 minutes)

Do all exercises listed below without stopping.

- ▼ **Regular jumping jacks: do as many as possible without stopping until 200**

- ▼ **Calf raises with finger flicks: 100 (without stopping)**

- ▼ **Calf stretch toe pulls: 10-count on each toe**

- ▼ **Gravity push-ups + superset w/regular push-ups: 10 reps, counting down from 10, 9, 8, etc., all the way down to 1. So:**

  10 gravity push-ups + 10 regular push-ups

  9 gravity push-ups + 9 regular push-ups

  And so on

- ▼ **Chest stretches: 10-count**

- ▼ **Shoulder boulders: 50-count**

- ▼ **Overhead arm pulls: 10 per side**

- ▼ **One-leg jumping jacks: 100 (straight) per leg**

30-second break.

Repeat.

TOUGH-LOVE TUESDAY
PHOTOS

Pictures of the following Tough-Love Tuesday exercises have already appeared:

- Jumping jack (page 35)

- Calf raise (page 36). To add "finger flicks," simply extend your arms out to your sides with a closed fist. Every time your heels go up, open your hands and fully extend your fingers. Close when your heels go down, then repeat.

- Calf stretch toe pull (page 21)

- Gravity push-up (page 42)

- Chest stretch (page 18)

- Overhead arm pull (page 16)

- One-leg jumping jack: do a regular jumping jack, but on one leg, simply hopping up and down on it while moving arms from sides to above your head and back

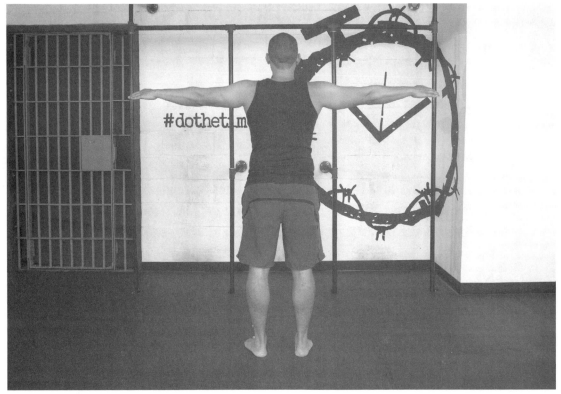

Shoulder boulder.
Standing, feet shoulder width apart. Hands directly by your side.
Bring both hands up so they connect with your shoulders. Then reach toward the back of your head and keep going until your hand reaches the opposite shoulder. Then bring it back to the same shoulder.
Then fully extend your arms out to your sides.

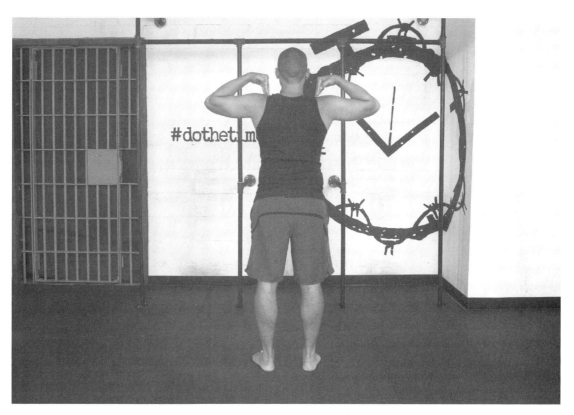

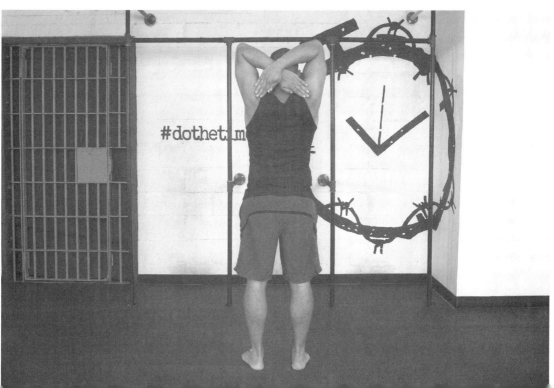

Lockdown Wednesday (30 minutes)

Leg Workout

Do all exercises listed below without stopping.

- ▼ Twisted jumping jacks: do as many as possible without stopping until 200

- ▼ Calf raises with finger flicks: 100 (without stopping)

- ▼ Calf stretch toe pulls: 10-count each toe

- ▼ High knees: 20

- ▼ Groin stretches (standing): 10-count per side

- ▼ Squat patties: 20

- ▼ Monkey F-ers: 20

- ▼ Quad stretches (lying down): 10-count per leg

- ▼ Lunge hops: 10 (if you need to take a break, do so—but then keep going)

- ▼ Leg lifts (lying down): 20

- ▼ Side leg raises: 20 per leg

- ▼ Butterfly stretches: 10-count

- ▼ Up-and-downs: 20

30-second break.

Repeat.

LOCKDOWN WEDNESDAY
PHOTOS

Pictures of the following Lockdown Wednesday exercises have already appeared:

- Twisted jumping jack (page 134)

- Calf raise (page 36). To add "finger flicks," simply extend your arms out to your sides with a closed fist. Every time your heels go up, open your hands and fully extend your fingers. Close when your heels go down, then repeat.

- Calf stretch toe pull (page 21)

- Groin stretch standing (page 27)

- Side leg raise (page 76)

- Butterfly stretch (page 24)

- Up-and-down (page 83)

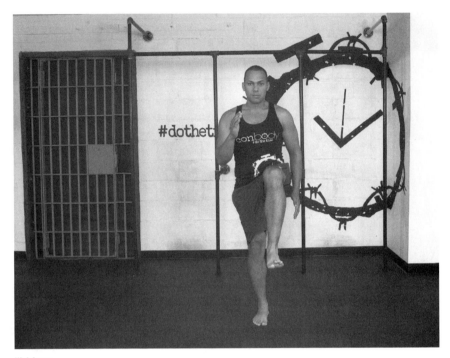

High knee.
Stand, feet shoulder width apart, hands by your side. Bring one knee just above your waist. Lower and repeat with opposite knee. Repeat, going back and forth.

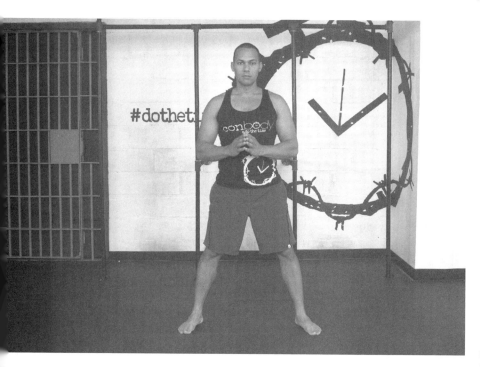

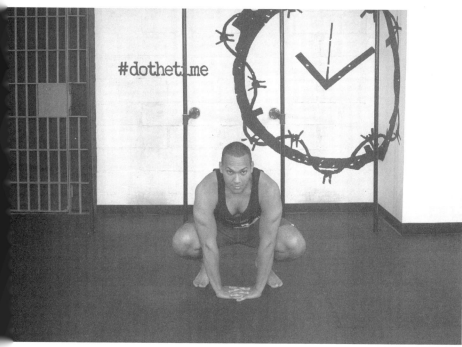

Squat patty.
Feet shoulder width apart, interlock fingers at chest. Lower palms to ground in a deep squat. Keep your feet flat on the ground. Then stand back up.

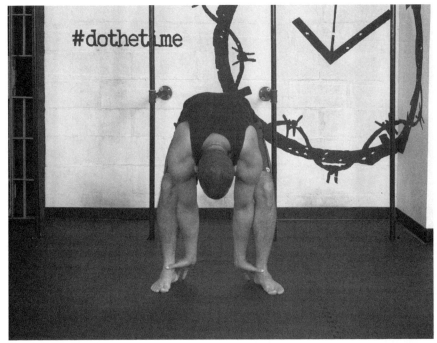

Monkey F-er.
Standing, extend your legs a little bit over shoulder width apart.
Keeping your heels on the ground, squat and lower both hands
so that you reach through the inside of your legs to
grab the back of your ankles.

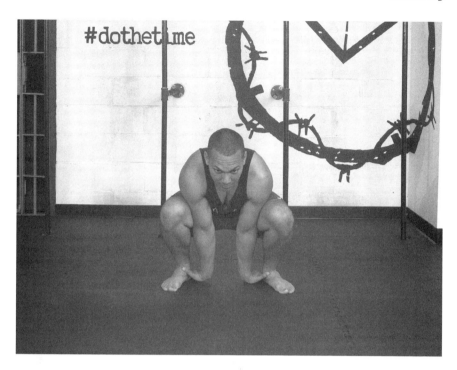

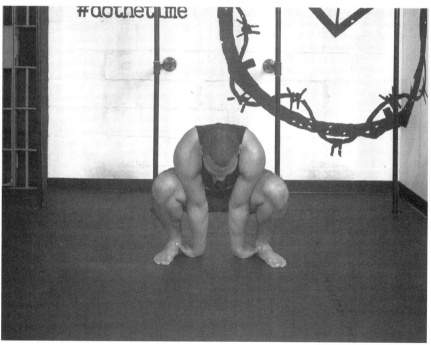

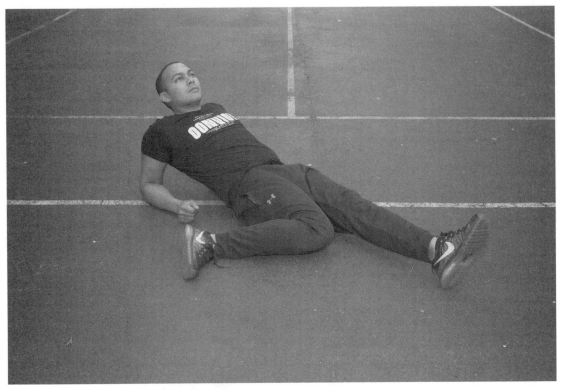

Quad stretch (lying down).
Lie down. Tuck one leg behind your butt. Leave the other fully extended forward. Lie back as far as you can. If you can't get down to your shoulder blades, rest on your elbows.

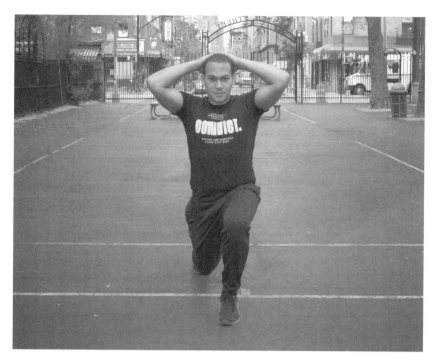

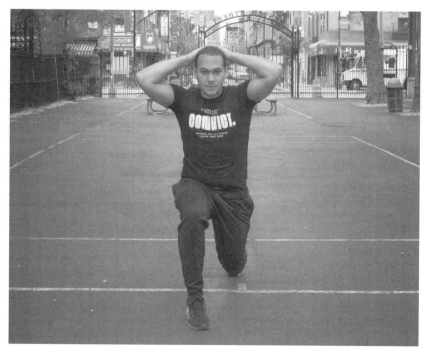

Lunge hop.

In lunge position, one knee on the ground at a 90-degree angle. Put your hands by the side of your head. Then hop up. While hopping, switch opposite knee down to the ground, bringing your other leg up to lunge.

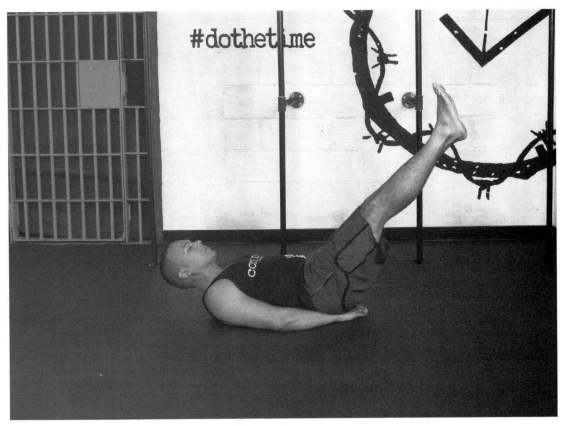

Leg lift.
Lie flat on your back, hands behind your butt, feet six inches off the ground. Raise your feet so your legs reach a 45-degree angle. Then bring them back to six inches. Then back up to 45 degrees. Repeat.

Hard-Core Thursday (30 minutes)

Core Workout

Do all exercises listed below without stopping.

▼ **Superset:**

50 jumping jacks (regular) + 50 plank jacks

40 jumping jacks (regular) + 40 plank jacks

30 jumping jacks (regular) + 30 plank jacks

20 jumping jacks (regular) + 20 plank jacks

10 jumping jacks (regular) + 10 plank jacks

▼ **Calf stretch toe pulls: 10-count on each toe**

▼ **Jumping jacks: 100 straight on each leg**

▼ **Abdominal stretches: 10-count**

▼ **3-minute abs (do as many as possible without legs down):**

30 supine bicycles

30 flutter kicks

30 scissor kicks

30 side-by-side twists

HARD-CORE THURSDAY
PHOTOS

Pictures of the following Hard-Core Thursday exercises have already appeared:

- Jumping jack (page 35)

- Calf stretch toe pull (page 21)

- Abdominal stretch (page 17)

- Supine bicycle (page 66)

- Flutter kick (page 70)

- Scissor kick (page 28)

- Side-by-side twist (page 68)

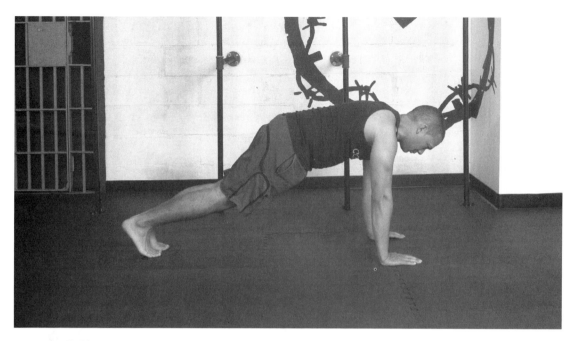

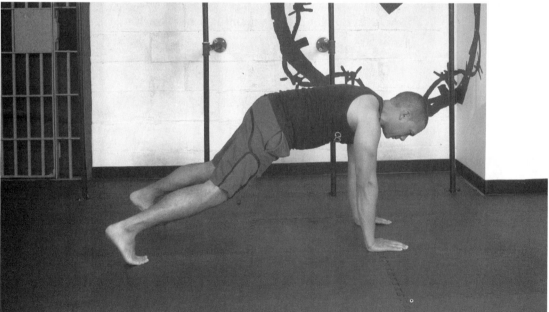

Plank jacks.
Get into push-up position, feet together, then open up legs like scissor jack and then close them back up.

Full-Body Friday (45 minutes)

Do all exercises listed below without stopping.

▼ **Squat-thrust countdown:**

   10 reps down to 1 rep, decreasing by 1 rep each set, taking
   5-second breaks between sets

▼ **Groin stretches (standing): 10-count per side**

▼ **Squat patties: 30 reps**

▼ **Hamstring stretches (standing): 10-count**

▼ **Monkey F-ers: 20 reps (by 4-count)**

▼ **Quad stretches (lying down): 10-count per leg**

▼ **Ski jumps: 30, side by side**

▼ **3-minute abs (do as many as possible without legs down):**

   30 supine bicycles

   30 flutter kicks

   30 scissor kicks

   30 side-by-side twists

▼ **10 to 1 countdown + superset:**

   Gravity push-ups (GPU) + regular push-ups (RPU)

       10 GPU reps + 10 RPU reps

       Repeat, decreasing by 1 rep each round,
       all the way down to 1

▼ **Overhead arm pulls: 10-count per arm**

FULL-BODY FRIDAY
PHOTOS

Pictures of the following Full-Body Friday exercises have already appeared:

- **Squat thrust (page 86)**

- **Groin stretch (standing) (page 27)**

- **Squat patty (page 143)**

- **Hamstring stretch (standing) (pages 22–23)**

- **Monkey F-er (page 144)**

- **Quad stretch (lying down) (page 146)**

- **Supine bicycle (page 66)**

- **Flutter kick (page 70)**

- **Scissor kick (page 28)**

- **Side-by-side twist (page 68)**

- **Gravity push-up (page 42)**

- **Overhead arm pull (page 16)**

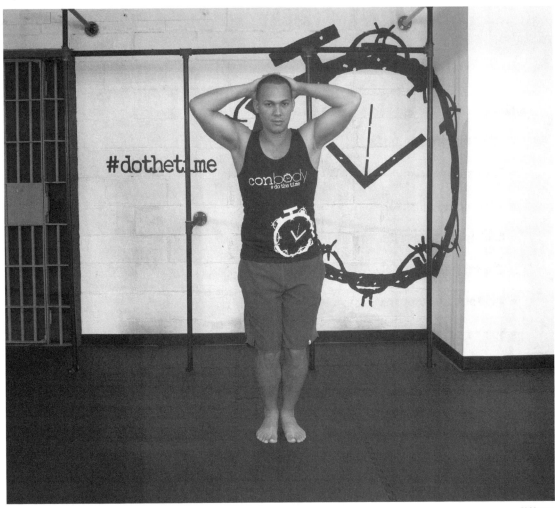

Ski jump.
Standing. Bring both feet together. Interlock hands on top of your head.
Keeping your feet together, jump to your side.
Then jump to your other side. Go back and forth, keeping feet together and hands locked on head.

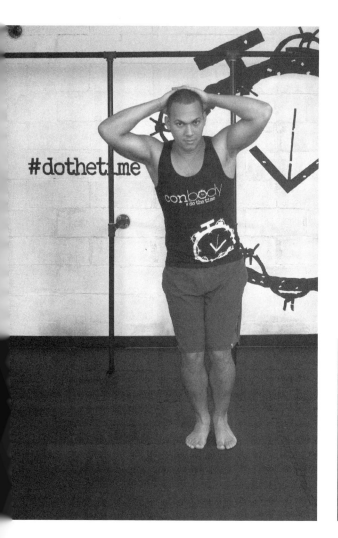
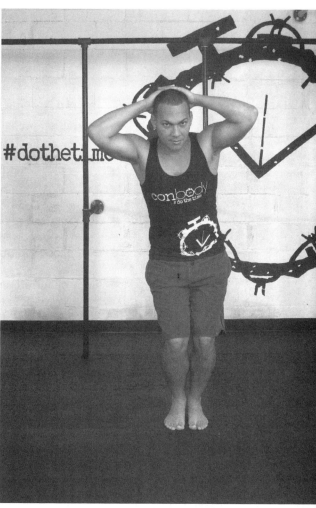

Superset Saturday (30 minutes)

Upper Body
Do all exercises listed below without stopping.

- ▼ Twisted jumping jacks: do as many as possible without stopping until 200

- ▼ Calf raises with finger flicks: 100-count without stopping

- ▼ Calf stretch toe pulls: 10-count on each toe

- ▼ Shoulder boulders: 50 reps

- ▼ Overhead arm pulls: 10-count per side

- ▼ 10 to 1 countdown + superset:

    Gravity push-ups (GPU) + regular push-ups (RPU)

    > 10 GPU reps + 10 RPU reps

    > Repeat, decreasing by 1 rep each round, all the way down to 1

- ▼ Toe touches: 30 per side

- ▼ T-bones: 30 reps

- ▼ Up-and-downs: 20 reps

- ▼ Chest stretches: 10-count

- ▼ Upper back stretches: 10 count

- ▼ Wing flaps: 100 reps

30-second break.

Repeat.

SUPERSET SATURDAY
PHOTOS

Pictures of the following Superset Saturday exercises have already appeared:

- Twisted jumping jack (page 134)

- Calf raise (page 36). To add "finger flicks," simply extend your arms out to your sides with a closed fist. Every time your heels go up, open your hands and fully extend your fingers.
  Close when your heels go down, then repeat.

- Calf stretch toe pull (page 21)

- Shoulder boulder (page 138)

- Overhead arm pull (page 16)

- Gravity push-up (page 42)

- Toe touch (page 79)

- T-bone (page 78)

- Up-and-down (page 83)

- Chest stretch (page 18)

- Upper back stretch (page 20)

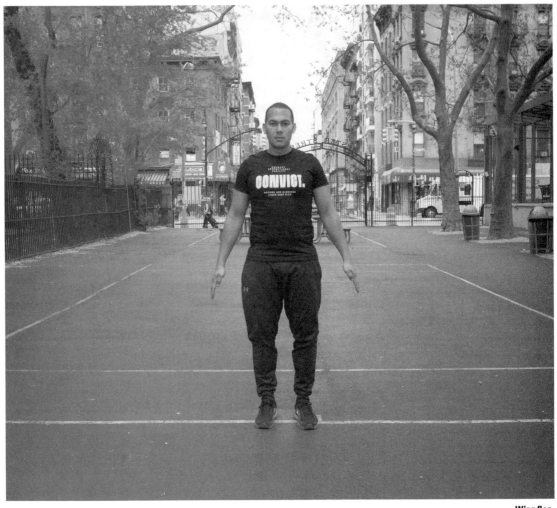

Wing flap.
Put your feet shoulder width apart, hands extended to side,
and bring hands down toward the side of your legs,
but without touching, and bring them back up and back down.

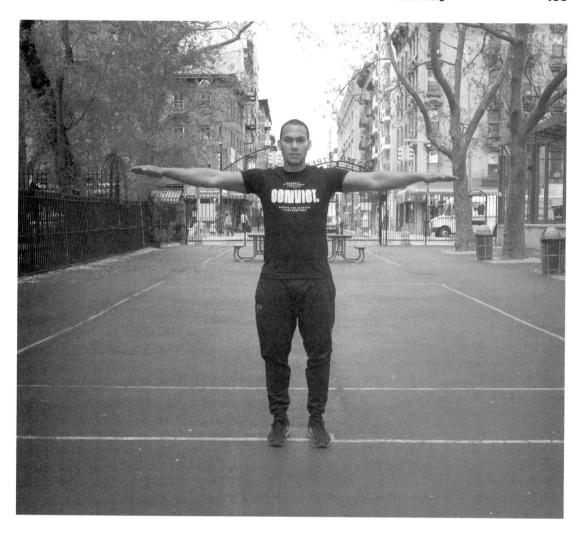

Slacking Sunday

Do all exercises listed below without stopping.

▼ **Rest**

▼ **Recover**

30-second break.

Repeat.

▼ **Relax and enjoy the day, so that you can do the time again in the new week.**

CONBODY BOOT CAMP
TWO MORE MONTHS

To take the ConBody boot-camp workout experience even further, here are two more weeks' worth of workouts that you can repeat for four weeks at a time, for a total of two months/sixty days more workout material.

(*REMINDER: When counting, count military style: one rep as "one-two-three-ONE," and so on.*)

From there, you can customize however you want using these exercises and/or others from throughout the book.

Whatever exercises you do, the most important thing will always be the following: Just do the time.

MONTH TWO
Repeat every week for four weeks.

Monday

Do all exercises listed below without stopping.

▼ **Around the World: 10 sets of each of the following, not stopping as long as possible. All of the equipment described in the following exercises may be found in your local park. If not, use the monkey bars in the child's playground for pull-ups.**

10 push-ups (any style)

Modify by putting your knees on the ground and leaning forward with your hands directly beneath your shoulders.

10 pull-ups

Modify by pulling yourself up over the bar, and holding for 10 seconds (or as long as possible).

10 dips

Modify by using a chair, bench, or ledge of any kind, instead of parallel bars.

MONTH TWO
MONDAY PHOTOS

Pictures of the following Around the World exercises have already appeared:

- Push-up (all styles) (starting on page 90)

- Pull-up (page 39)

- Dip (page 37)

Tuesday

Do all exercises listed below without stopping.

- ▼ **Regular jumping jacks: 50**

- ▼ **Squat patties: 30**

- ▼ **Heel touches: 40 per side**

- ▼ **Lunges: 20 per leg**

- ▼ **High knees: 30**

- ▼ **Back and forths: 15**

- ▼ **Up-and-downs: 20**

- ▼ **Squat hold: 30 seconds**

- ▼ **Squat jumps: 30**

- ▼ **Squat hold: 10 seconds**

- ▼ **Up-and-downs: 10**

- ▼ **Side leg raises: 20 per side**

- ▼ **Flutter kicks: 40**

- ▼ **Side-by-side twists: 30**

- ▼ **Scissor kicks: 20**

- ▼ **Supine bicycles: 10**

20–30-second break, sip of water.

▼ **Prison Baseball**

In a nine-by-six-foot space (the size of a cell, or small living room), do 8–10 laps around or 4–5 laps back and forth:

> First Lap

>> Lunge walk

>> Lunge hops: 20 each knee

>> Pull-up bar: 10-second hold

> Second Lap

>> Bear crawl

>> Mountain climbers: 20-count

>> Pull-up bar: 10-second hold

> Third Lap

>> Gorilla walk

>> Monkey F-ers: 40

>> Pull-up bar: 10-second hold

> Fourth Lap

>> Crab walk

>> Toe touches: 10

>> Pull-up bar: 10-second hold

> Fifth Lap

>> Push-up walk

>> Squat hold: 60 seconds

>> Pull-up bar: 10-second hold

MONTH TWO
TUESDAY PHOTOS

Pictures of the following Month Two (Tuesday) exercises have already appeared:

- Jumping jack (page 35)

- Squat patty (page 143)

- Lunge (page 88)

- High knee (page 142)

- Back and forth (page 80)

- Up-and-down (page 83)

- Side leg raise (page 76)

- Flutter kick (page 70)

- Side-by-side twist (page 68)

- Scissor kick (page 28)

- Supine bicycle (page 66)

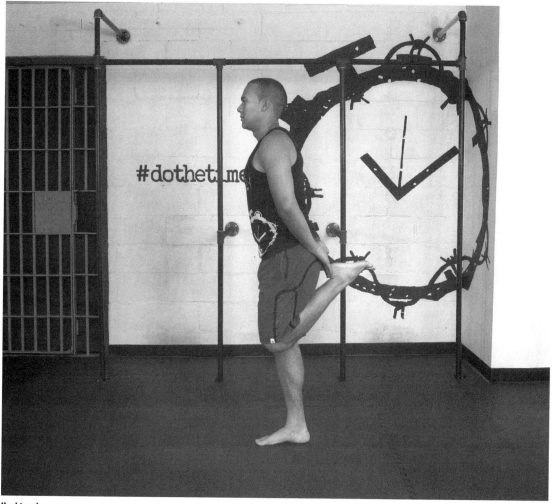

Heel touch.
Standing with your feet side by side, kick one heel up to your butt and tap it with your fingers on the same hand side, take it
back down to the floor, then repeat with the other foot, and so on. Sort of like running in place.

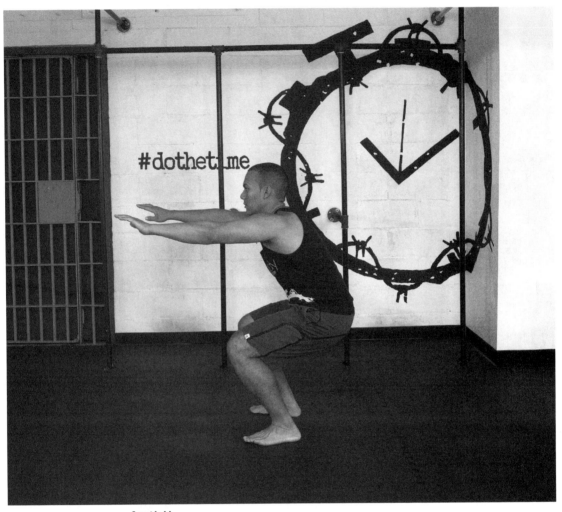

Squat hold.
From standing position, go into a squat so your knees are almost 90 degrees. Hold.

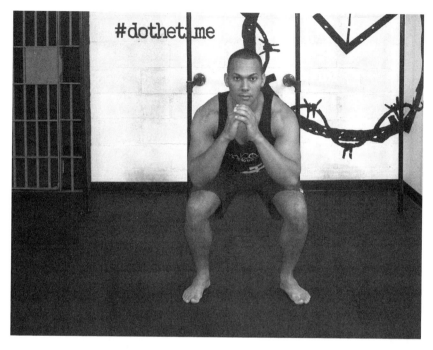

Squat jump.
Stand up straight. Then squat. Then jump straight up high as you can. Repeat.

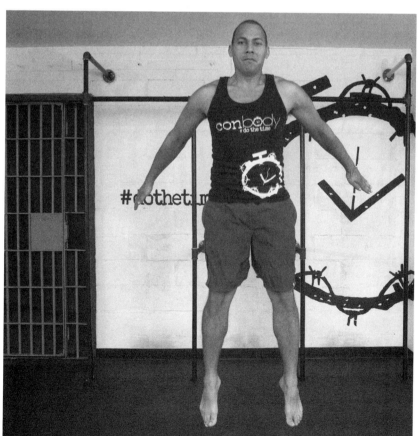

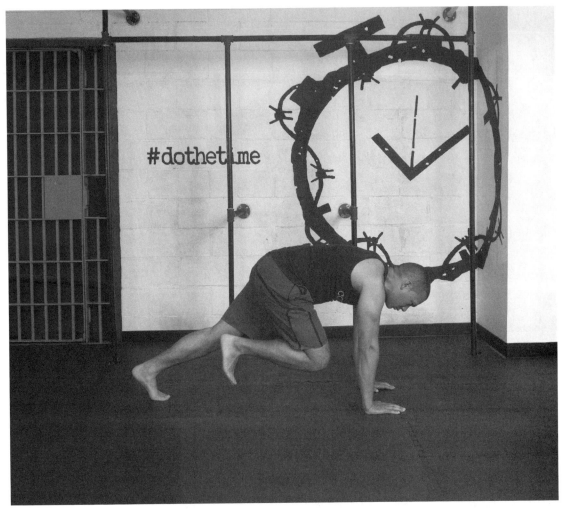

Mountain climber.

Start in push-up position, arms extended with hands shoulder-width apart on the ground.

Bring one foot forward so that your knee tucks up into your chest, then extend foot back and place on the ground. Then quickly do the same with your opposite foot. And repeat.

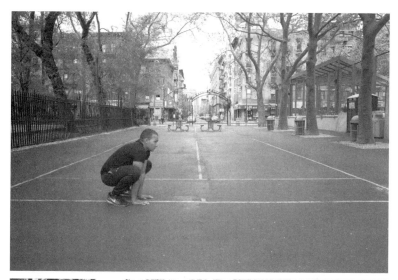

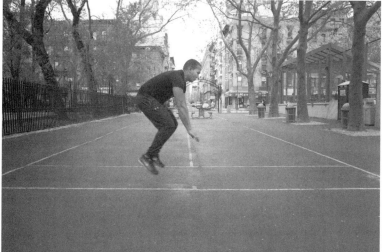

Gorilla walk.

Squat so that your hands are on the ground between your legs, a little less than shoulder-width apart. You should be on the balls of your feet or your tiptoes. Extend both hands forward at the same time, as far as you can, and after your hands land, bring both feet forward at the same time, to catch up to your hands. Repeat.

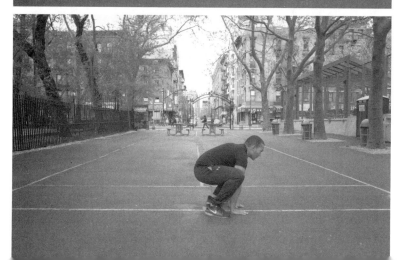

Prison Baseball

Pictures of the following Prison Baseball exercises have already appeared:

- Lunge walk (page 104)

- Lunge hop (page 147)

- Pull-up (hold) (page 39)

- Bear crawl (page 102)

- Monkey F-er (page 144)

- Crab walk (page 62)

- Toe touch (page 79)

- Push-up walk (page 98)

- Squat hold (page 168)

Wednesday

Do all exercises listed below without stopping.

▼ **Around the World: 10 sets of each of the following, not stopping as long as possible. All of the equipment described in the following exercises may be found in your local park. If not, use the monkey bars in the child's playground for pull-ups.**

10 push-ups (any style)

> *Modify by putting your knees on the ground and leaning forward with your hands directly beneath your shoulders.*

10 chin-ups

> *Modify by pulling yourself up over the bar, and holding for 10 seconds (or as long as possible).*

10 dips

> *Modify by using a chair, bench, or ledge of any kind, instead of parallel bars.*

MONTH TWO
WEDNESDAY PHOTOS

Pictures of the following Around the World exercises have already appeared:

- Push-up (all styles) (starting on page 90)

- Chin-up (page 40)

- Dip (page 37)

Thursday

Do all exercises listed below without stopping.

- ▼ Regular jumping jacks: 50
- ▼ Plank jacks: 30
- ▼ Heel touches: 40
- ▼ Mountain climbers: 20
- ▼ High knees: 30
- ▼ Plank climbers crawl (in place): 15
- ▼ Squat thrusts: 20
- ▼ Up-and-downs: 10
- ▼ Push-up plank: 50 seconds
- ▼ Plank jacks: 20-count
- ▼ Plank: 30 seconds
- ▼ Lay-up-and-down: 20-count
- ▼ Push-ups: 10 (all the way down, no knees)

Stand up.

- ▼ Up-and-downs: 10
- ▼ Six inches: 50 seconds
- ▼ Flutter kicks: 40
- ▼ Sit-ups: 30
- ▼ Scissor kicks: 20
- ▼ Supine bicycles: 10

20–30-second break, sip of water.

▼ **Prison Baseball:**

In a nine-by-six-foot space (the size of a cell, or small living room), do 8–10 laps around or 4–5 laps back and forth:

First Lap

Lunge walk

Lunge hops: 20 each knee

Pull-up bar: 10-second hold

Second Lap

Bear crawl

Mountain climbers: 20-count

Pull-up bar: 10-second hold

Third Lap

Gorilla walk

Monkey F-ers: 40

Pull-up bar: 10-second hold

Fourth Lap

Crab walk

Toe touches: 10

Pull-up bar: 10-second hold

Fifth Lap

Push-up walk

Squat hold: 60 seconds

Pull-up bar: 10-second hold

MONTH TWO
THURSDAY PHOTOS

Pictures of the following Month Two (Thursday) exercises can be found earlier:

- Jumping jack (page 35)

- Plank jack (page 151)

- Heel touch (page 167)

- Mountain climber 170)

- High knee (page 142)

- Squat thrust (page 86)

- Up-and-down (page 83)

- Plank (page 75)

- Lay-up-and-down (page 65)

- Push-up (page [90)

- Flutter kick (page 70)

- Sit-up (page 44)

- Scissor kick (page 28)

- Supine bicycle (page 66)

Prison Baseball

Pictures of the following Prison Baseball exercises have already appeared:

- **Lunge walk (page 104)**

- **Lunge hop (page 147)**

- **Pull-up (hold) (page 39)**

- **Bear crawl (page 102)**

- **Mountain climber (page 170)**

- **Gorilla walk (page 171)**

- **Monkey F-er (page 144)**

- **Crab walk (page 62)**

- **Toe touch (page 79)**

- **Push-up walk (page 98)**

- **Squat hold (page 168)**

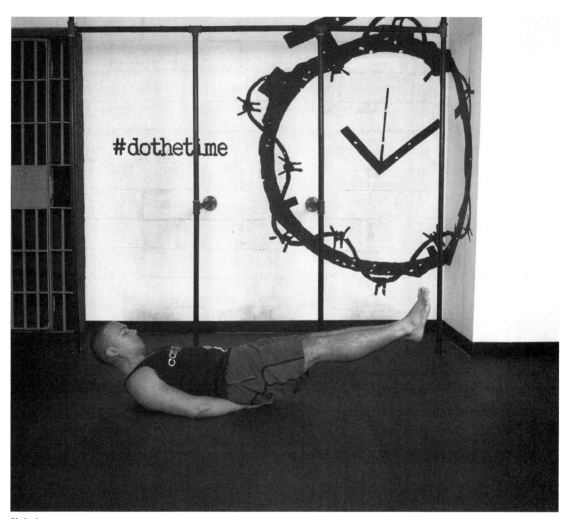

Six inches.
Lie flat on back. Tuck your hands under your lower back/butt.
Keeping legs locked out, raise feet about six inches off the ground. Hold.

Friday

▼ **Around the World: 10 sets of each of the following, not stopping as long as possible. All of the equipment described in the following exercises may be found in your local park. If not, use the monkey bars in the child's playground for pull-ups.**

10 push-ups (any style)

Modify by putting your knees on the ground and leaning forward with your hands directly beneath your shoulders.

10 pull-ups

Modify by pulling yourself up over the bar, and holding for 10 seconds (or as long as possible).

10 dips

Modify by using a chair, bench, or ledge of any kind, instead of parallel bars.

MONTH TWO
FRIDAY PHOTOS

Pictures of the following Around the World exercises have already appeared:

- Push-up (all styles) (starting on page 90)

- Pull-up (page 39)

- Dip (page 37)

Saturday

Do all exercises listed below without stopping.

- ▼ **Regular jumping jacks: 50**

- ▼ **Plank jacks: 30**

- ▼ **Heel touches: 40**

- ▼ **Mountain climbers: 20**

- ▼ **High knees: 30**

- ▼ **Plank climbers crawl: 15**

- ▼ **Squat thrusts: 20**

- ▼ **Up-and-downs: 10**

- ▼ **Push-up plank: 50 seconds**

- ▼ **Plank jacks: 20-count**

- ▼ **Lay-up-and-down: 20-count**

- ▼ **Push-ups: 10 (all the way down, no knees)**

  Stand up.

- ▼ **Up-and-downs: 10**

- ▼ **Six inches: 50 seconds**

- ▼ **Flutter kicks: 40**

- ▼ **Sit-ups: 30**

- ▼ **Scissor kicks: 20**

- ▼ **Supine bicycles: 10**

20–30-second break, sip of water.

▼ **Prison Baseball:**

In a nine-by-six-foot space (the size of a cell, or small living room), do 8–10 laps around or 4–5 laps back and forth:

    First Lap

            Lunge walk

            Lunge hops: 20 each knee

            Pull-up bar: 10-second hold

    Second Lap

            Bear crawl

            Mountain climbers: 20-count

            Pull-up bar: 10-second hold

    Third Lap

            Gorilla walk

            Monkey F-ers: 40

            Pull-up bar: 10-second hold

    Fourth Lap

            Crab walk

            Toe touches: 10

            Pull-up bar: 10-second hold

    Fifth Lap

            Push-up walk

            Squat hold: 60 seconds

            Pull-up bar: 10-second hold

MONTH TWO
SATURDAY PHOTOS

Pictures of the following Month Two (Saturday) exercises have already appeared:

- Jumping jack (page 35)

- Plank jack (page 151)

- Heel touch (page 167)

- Mountain climber (page 170)

- High knee (page 142)

- Plank climbers crawl (in place) (page 100)

- Squat thrust (page 86)

- Up-and-down (page 83)

- Push-up plank: do push-up (page 90),
  then hold plank position for 30 seconds

- Lay-up-and-down (page 65)

- Push-up (page 90)

- Six inches (page 179)

- Flutter kick (page 70)

- Sit-up (page 44)

- Scissor kick (page 28)

- Supine bicycle (page 66)

Prison Baseball

Pictures of the following Prison Baseball exercises have already appeared:

- Lunge walk (page 104)

- Lunge hop (page 147)

- Pull-up (hold) (page 39)

- Bear crawl (page 102)

- Mountain climber (page 170)

- Gorilla walk (page 171)

- Monkey F-er (page 144)

- Crab walk (page 62)

- Toe touch (page 79)

- Push-up walk (page 98)

- Squat hold (page 168)

Sunday

Recovery Day.

Or...

▼ **Around the World: 10 sets of each of the following, not stopping as long as possible. All of the equipment described in the following exercises may be found in your local park. If not, use the monkey bars in the child's playground for pull-ups.**

10 push-ups (any style)

Modify by putting your knees on the ground and leaning forward with your hands directly beneath your shoulders.

10 pull-ups

Modify by pulling yourself up over the bar, and holding for 10 seconds (or as long as possible).

10 dips

Modify by using a chair, bench, or ledge of any kind, instead of parallel bars.

MONTH TWO
SUNDAY PHOTOS

Pictures of the following Around the World exercises have already appeared:

- Push-up (all styles) (starting on page 90)

- Pull-up (page 39)

- Dip (page 37)

CONBODY BOOT CAMP
MONTH THREE

Repeat every week for four weeks.

Monday

Do all exercises listed below without stopping.

▼ **Regular jumping jacks: 50**

▼ **Plank jacks: 30**

▼ **Heel touches: 40**

▼ **Mountain climbers: 20**

▼ **High knees: 30**

▼ **Plank climbers crawl: 15**

▼ **Squat thrusts: 20**

▼ **Up-and-downs: 10**

▼ **Push-up plank: 50 seconds**

▼ **Plank jacks: 20-count**

▼ **Plank: 30 seconds**

▼ **Lay-up-and-down: 20-count**

▼ **Push-ups: 10 (all the way down, no knees)**

Stand up.

▼ **Up-and-downs:** 10

▼ **Six inches:** 50 seconds

▼ **Flutter kicks:** 40

▼ **Sit-ups:** 30

▼ **Scissor kicks:** 20

▼ **Supine bicycles:** 10

20–30-second break, sip of water.

▼ **Prison Baseball:**

In a nine-by-six-foot space (the size of a cell, or small living room), do 8–10 laps around or 4–5 laps back and forth:

First Lap

Lunge walk

Lunge hops: 20 each knee

Pull-up bar: 10-second hold

Second Lap

Bear crawl

Mountain climbers: 20-count

Pull-up bar: 10-second hold

Third Lap

Gorilla walk

Monkey F-ers: 40

Pull-up bar: 10-second hold

Fourth Lap

Crab walk

Toe touches: 10

Pull-up bar: 10-second hold

Fifth Lap

Push-up walk

Squat hold: 60 seconds

Pull-up bar: 10-second hold

MONTH THREE
MONDAY PHOTOS

Pictures of the following Month Three (Monday) exercises have already appeared:

- **Jumping jack (page 35)**

- **Plank jack (page 151)**

- **Heel touch (page 167)**

- **Mountain climbers (page 170)**

- **High knees (page 142)**

- **Plank climbers crawl (page 100)**

- **Squat thrust (page 86)**

- **Up-and-down (page 83)**

- **Push-up plank: do push-up (page 90) then hold plank position for 30 seconds**

- **Plank (page 75)**

- **Push-up (page 90)**

- **Six inches (page 179)**

- **Flutter kick (page 70)**

- **Sit-up (page 44)**

- **Scissor kick (page 28)**

- **Supine bicycle (page 66)**

Prison Baseball

Pictures of the following Prison Baseball exercises have already appeared:

- Lunge walk (page 104)

- Lunge hop (page 147)

- Pull-up (hold) (page 39)

- Bear crawl (page 102)

- Mountain climber (page 170)

- Gorilla walk (page 171)

- Monkey F-er (page 144)

- Crab walk (page 62)

- Toe touch (page 79)

- Push-up walk (page 98)

- Squat hold (page 168)

Tuesday

Do all exercises listed below without stopping.

- ▼ Twisted jumping jacks: 50-count

- ▼ Push-up plank: 100 seconds

- ▼ Heel touches: 40-count

- ▼ Plank: 60 seconds

- ▼ High knee: 30

- ▼ Plank climbers crawl: 15

- ▼ Squat thrusts: 20

- ▼ Up-and-downs: 10

- ▼ Push-up plank: 50 seconds

- ▼ Regular push-ups: 20

- ▼ Plank: 30 seconds

- ▼ Lay-up-and-down: 20-count

- ▼ Push-ups: 10 (all the way down, no knees, try your best always)

Stand up.

- ▼ Up-and-downs: 20

- ▼ Six inches: 100 seconds

- ▼ Crunches: 20-count

- ▼ Flutter kicks: 30-count

▼ Scissor kicks: 20

▼ Supine bicycles: 10

20–30-second break, sip of water.

▼ Exercise Laps

These are laps around a nine-by-six-foot space (the size of a cell, or small living room)

First Lap

Lunge walk: 2 steps forward, then backward 5 laps

Lunge hops: 10 each side

Second Lap

Bear crawl: 2 steps forward, then backward 4 laps

Mountain climbers: 20-count

Third Lap

Gorilla walk: 2 steps forward, then backward 3 laps

Monkey F-ers: 40

Fourth Lap

Crab walk: 2 steps forward, then backward 2 laps

Toe touches: 10

Fifth Lap

Push-up walk: 5 steps forward, then backward 1 lap

Push-up plank: 60-second hold

MONTH THREE
TUESDAY PHOTOS

Pictures of the following Month Three (Tuesday) exercises have already appeared:

- Twisted jumping jack (page 134)

- Push-up plank: do push-up (page 90),
  then hold plank position for 30 seconds

- Heel touch (page 167)

- High knee (page 142)

- Plank climbers crawl (page 100)

- Squat thrust (page 86)

- Up-and-down (page 83)

- Push-up (page 90)

- Plank (page 75)

- Lay-up-and-down (page 65)

- Six inches (page 179)

- Crunch (page 74)

- Flutter kick (page 70)

- Scissor kick (page 28)

- Supine bicycle (page 66)

Exercise Laps

Pictures of the following Exercise Laps have already appeared:

- Lunge walk (page 104)

- Lunge hop (page 147)

- Bear crawl (page 102)

- Mountain climber (page 170)

- Gorilla walk (page 171)

- Monkey F-er (page 144)

- Crab walk (page 62)

- Toe touch (page 79)

- Push-up walk (page 98)

- Push-up plank: do push-Up (page [90),
  then hold plank position for 60 seconds

Wednesday

Do all exercises listed below without stopping.

▼ **Regular jumping jacks: 50**

▼ **Squat patties: 30**

▼ **Heel touches: 40**

▼ **Lunges: 20 per leg**

▼ **High knees: 30**

▼ **T-bones: 15**

▼ **Up-and-downs: 20**

▼ **Squat hold: 30 seconds**

▼ **Squat thrusts: 50**

▼ **Squat hold: 10 seconds**

▼ **Up-and-downs: 10**

▼ **Side leg raises: 20 per side**

▼ **Flutter kicks: 40**

▼ **Sit-ups: 30**

▼ **Scissor kicks: 20**

▼ **Supine bicycles: 10**

20–30-second break, sip of water.

▼ **Prison Baseball**

In a nine-by-six-foot space (the size of a cell, or small living room), do 8–10 laps around or 4–5 laps back and forth:

First Lap

    Lunge walk

    Lunge hops: 20 each knee

    Pull-up bar: 10-second hold

Second Lap

    Bear crawl

    Mountain climbers: 20-count

    Pull-up bar: 10-second hold

Third Lap

    Gorilla walk

    Monkey F-ers: 40

    Pull-up bar: 10-second hold

Fourth Lap

    Crab walk

    Toe touches: 10

    Pull-up bar: 10-second hold

Fifth Lap

    Push-up walk

    Squat hold: 60 seconds

    Pull-up bar: 10-second hold

MONTH THREE
WEDNESDAY PHOTOS

Pictures of the following Month Three (Wednesday) exercises have already appeared:

- Jumping jack (page 35)

- Squat patty (page 143)

- Heel touch (page 167)

- Lunge (page 88)

- High knee (page 142)

- T-bone (page 78)

- Up-and-down (page 83)

- Squat hold (page 168)

- Squat thrust (page 86)

- Side leg raise (page 76)

- Flutter kick (page 70)

- Sit-up (page 44)

- Scissor kick (page 28)

- Supine bicycle (page 66)

Prison Baseball

Pictures of the following Prison Baseball exercises have already appeared:

- Lunge walk (page 104)

- Lunge hop (page 147)

- Pull-up (hold) (page 39)

- Bear crawl (page 102)

- Mountain climber (page 170)

- Gorilla walk (page 171)

- Monkey F-er (page 144)

- Crab walk (page 62)

- Toe touch (page 79)

- Push-up walk (page 98)

- Squat hold (page 168)

Thursday

Do all exercises listed below without stopping.

▼ Regular jumping jacks: 50

▼ Plank jacks: 30

▼ Heel touches: 40

▼ Mountain climbers: 20

▼ High knees: 30

▼ Plank climbers crawl (in place): 15

▼ Squat thrusts: 20

▼ Up-and-downs: 10

▼ Push-up plank: 50 seconds

▼ Plank jacks: 20-count

▼ Plank: 30 seconds

▼ Lay-up-and-down: 20-count

▼ Push-ups: 10 (all the way down, no knees)

Stand up.

▼ Up-and-downs: 10

▼ Six inches: 50 seconds

▼ Flutter kicks: 40

▼ Sit-ups: 30

▼ **Scissor kicks: 20**

▼ **Supine bicycles: 10**

20–30-second break, sip of water.

▼ **Exercise Laps**

These are laps around a nine-by-six-foot space
(the size of a cell, or small living room)

First Lap

Bear crawl: 2 steps forward,
then backward 4 laps

Mountain climbers: 20-count

Second Lap

Crab walk: 2 steps forward,
then backward 2 laps

Toe touches: 10

Third Lap

Gorilla walk: 2 steps forward,
then backward 3 laps

Monkey F-ers: 40

Fourth Lap

Plank climbers crawl: 5 steps forward,
then backward 1 lap

Push-up plank: 60-second hold

Fifth Lap

Push-up walk: 5 steps forward,
then backward 1 lap

Regular push-ups: 20

MONTH THREE
THURSDAY PHOTOS

Pictures of the following Month Three (Thursday) exercises have already appeared:

- Jumping jack (page 35)

- Plank jack (page 151)

- Heel touch (page 167)

- Mountain climber (page 170)

- High knee (page 142)

- Plank climbers crawl (in place) (page 100)

- Squat thrust (page 86)

- Up-and-down (page 83)

- Push-up plank: do push-up (page 90),
  then hold plank position for 30 seconds

- Plank (page [75)

- Lay-up-and-down (page 65)

- Push-ups (page 90)

- Six inches (page 179)

- Flutter kick (page 70)

- Sit-up (page 44)

- Scissor kick (page 28)

- Supine bicycle (page 66)

Exercise Laps

Pictures of the following Exercise Laps have already appeared:

- Bear crawl (page 102)

- Mountain climber (page 170)

- Crab walk (page 62)

- Toe touch (page 79)

- Gorilla walk (page 171)

- Monkey F-er (page 144)

- Plank climbers crawl (in place) (page 100)

- Push-up plank: do push-up (page 90), then hold plank position for 30 seconds

- Push-up walk (page 98)

- Push-ups (page 90)

Friday

Do all exercises listed below without stopping.

▼ **Regular jumping jacks: 50**

▼ **Squat thrusts: 30**

▼ **Heel touches: 40**

▼ **Squat thrusts: 20**

▼ **High knees: 30**

▼ **Squat thrusts: 15**

▼ **Body builders: 20**

10-second break.

▼ **Body builders: 15**

10-second break.

▼ **Body builders: 10**

10-second break.

▼ **Squat jumps: 50**

▼ **Squat hold: 20 seconds**

▼ **Squat jumps: 30**

▼ **Squat hold: 10 seconds**

▼ **Up-and-downs: 10**

▼ **Side leg raises: 20 per side**

▼ **Flutter kicks: 40**

▼ **Sit-ups: 30-count**

▼ **Scissor kicks: 20**

▼ **Supine bicycles: 10**

20–30-second break, sip of water.

▼ **Prison Baseball**

In a nine-by-six-foot space (the size of a cell, or small living room), do 8–10 laps around or 4–5 laps back and forth:

First Lap

Lunge walk

Lunge hops: 20 each knee

Pull-up bar: 10-second hold

Second Lap

Bear crawl

Mountain climbers: 20-count

Pull-up bar: 10-second hold

Third Lap

Gorilla walk

Monkey F-ers: 40

Pull-up bar: 10-second hold

Fourth Lap

Crab walk

Toe touch: 10

Pull-up bar: 10-second hold

Fifth Lap

Push-up walk

Squat hold: 60 seconds

Pull-up bar: 10-second hold

MONTH THREE
FRIDAY PHOTOS

Pictures of the following Month Three (Friday) exercises have already appeared:

- Jumping jack (page 35)

- Squat thrust (page 86)

- Heel touch (page 167)

- High knee (page 142)

- Squat jump (page 169)

- Squat hold (page 168)

- Up-and-down (page 83)

- Side leg raise (page 76)

- Flutter kick (page 70)

- Sit-up (page 44)

- Scissor kick (page 28)

- Supine bicycle (page 66)

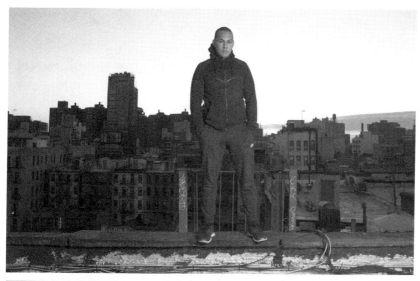

Body builders.

This is an eight-count movement. Begin by standing with both feet together, hands by your side. Proceed quickly.

On one: Squat and place your hands on the ground.

Two: Kick your legs straight back, so that you move into a push-up position.

Three: Kick your feet out so they land about shoulder-width apart, while holding the push-up position (like the plank jack).

Four: Bring your feet back together.

Five and six: Lower your body to the ground (on five) then do a push-up (on six).

Seven: Tuck your feet back up under you so that you are back in a squatting position.

Eight: Stand up straight.

And repeat.

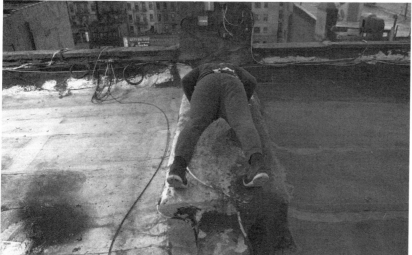

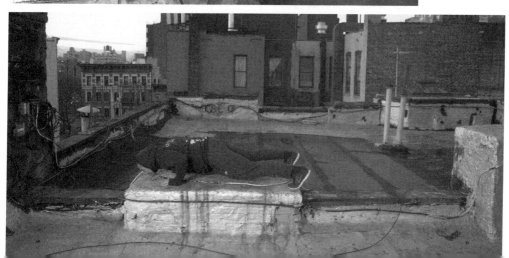

Prison Baseball

Pictures of the following Prison Baseball exercises have already appeared:

- Lunge walk (page 104)

- Lunge hop (page 147)

- Pull-up (hold) (page 39)

- Bear crawl (page 102)

- Mountain climber (page 170)

- Gorilla walk (page 171)

- Monkey F-er (page 144)

- Crab walk (page 62)

- Toe touch (page 79)

- Push-up walk (page 98)

- Squat hold (page 168)

Saturday

Do all exercises listed below without stopping.

▼ **Around the World: 10 sets of each of the following, not stopping as long as possible. All of the equipment described in the following exercises may be found in your local park. If not, use the monkey bars in the child's playground for pull-ups.**

10 push-ups (any style)

Modify by putting your knees on the ground and leaning forward with your hands directly beneath your shoulders.

10 pull-ups

Modify by pulling yourself up over the bar, and holding for 10 seconds (or as long as possible).

10 dips

Modify by using a chair, bench, or ledge of any kind, instead of parallel bars.

MONTH THREE
SATURDAY PHOTOS

Pictures of the following Around the World exercises have already appeared:

- Push-up (all styles) (starting on page 90)

- Pull-up (page 39)

- Dip (page 37)

Sunday

▼ Rest.

FINAL NOTE

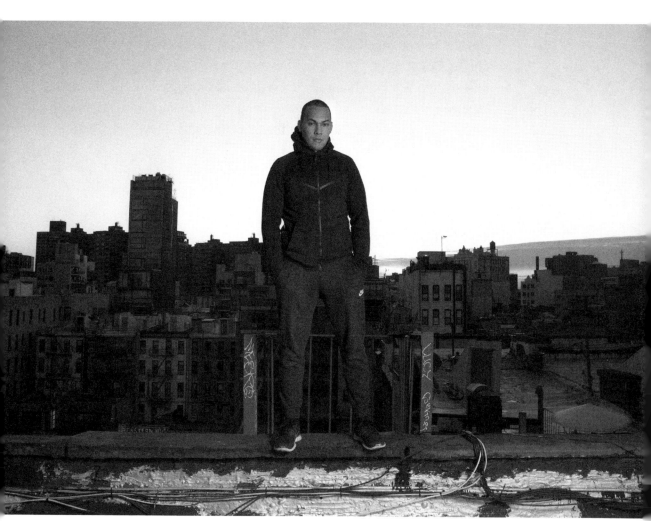

Standing on the roof of my building at the corner of Broome and Eldridge, where it all began, where it all ended, and where it's all begun again. Hard to believe I'm here. Took a lot of hard work, but it's worth it. I'm free.

Ten years ago, when I was a kid, I never believed that anybody from my neighborhood could stay there and become something like what I've become today. I'm not bragging. I'm in shock about it. I've gone from convicted drug kingpin to successful businessman—successful enough that the world's biggest media companies, from BuzzFeed to Bleacher Report to *The New York Times*—have covered me, my story, and the ConBody movement, and all that has happened right here in my Lower East Side neighborhood. Some days, I still can't believe it's real. If I'd seen someone like me back when I was a kid, I still wouldn't have believed it was actually possible. I would have thought that person was super rare, and super lucky, and that there was no way anyone else could do that.

I am lucky.

And maybe I am rare.

But I am not unique.

I am not an aberration.

I mean this both inspirationally and practically.

|||||||||

First, the practical: I have placed my faith in others like myself, and seen that faith rewarded.

Remember the soul of the workout—that hard, simple thing to grasp:

Just do the time.

I said it at the start, and I'll say it here again: These workouts will change your life if you let them.

That sounds dramatic, but I guess sometimes the truth is dramatic. As you've gotten to know me throughout this book, I hope you've seen just how undramatic I am. This book could have been twice as long and looked way more impressive if I'd made it the length my publisher originally put in our contract. My cowriter and I convinced them to keep it short, to cut the fat—to cut the unnecessary drama. The message is too important to get lost in drama.

Drama is good sometimes, because it gets your attention.

But sometimes, like grease or sugar or Prison Burritos, it's just another distraction—something we think keeps us sane, but really makes us more insane.

To feel dramatic feels good.

And yeah, drama is some addictive shit.

It can wreck you easy as any drug.

Which brings me to the faith I placed in others, and the rewards that faith has reaped.

IIIIIIII

Again, I want to say that if you are in a prison, then this is for you. Maybe your prison is the type with iron bars and stone walls with razor wire on top. Maybe your prison is a hundred pounds of fat. Maybe both. Maybe something else: alcohol, weed, fatty food. Maybe it's all of the above, and more.

The world is full of things that can lock us up.

And the world is full of people waiting to convince you that you can never be free.

And in the battle between our humanity and our fear, it is so easy to let fear win.

Human beings are wired to improve—to improve themselves, to improve each other, to improve the world.

When that wiring is hijacked, when we find ourselves addicted to the wrong things, is when we start to die.

And an addiction equally as destructive as any substance is an addiction to what other people think of us.

So I know how you feel when people look at you and don't see you for who you know yourself to be in your heart. It makes you feel hopeless and the next thing you know, you're reverting back to old patterns just because that's what you knew to do to survive. That's what you knew to do so you could feel safe and comfortable.

I get it.

It's human.

You're human.

But I also want you to know something.

I know this because I am free, but also because of the people I've seen set free along with me.

The world's perception of you doesn't matter.

If you're happy with who you are, then be happy and f--k the world.

But if you want to change it, then you can. It is possible.

I speak from what I have witnessed with my workout clients. But I also speak from what I have seen with my ConBody employees.

It's the same battle faced by those of us coming out of literal prisons, too.

Same as when I was fat running around the yard getting mocked and yelled at by those guys on S-Block—*"Run, run, Honey Bun!"* When I got out of prison and people learned I was an ex-con, I felt a different sort of judgment. It's the same judgment all of us who've done time feel. People see us ex-cons in a dramatically different way than anyone else—especially us ex-cons of color.

I have about twenty staff members as of this writing—and almost all of them are ex-cons. Almost all of them are felons. Almost all of them couldn't find work anywhere else.

Same as the way I developed my unhealthy diet and lifestyle that made me fat and shot my blood pressure and cholesterol into the stratosphere, the same is true of us who become criminals:

The reasons we were first imprisoned weren't because we were bad people trying to do bad things, but because we came from places that taught us lessons that were simply wrong. And we did not know better until it was too late.

I know a lot of felons and most of them are not purely bad people at heart—in their hearts most of them are good people who did bad things, and want to make those things right. Most are people who, like all of us, came to believe certain things were a certain way when they were young. By the time we were old enough to understand reality, we had already made mistakes. Yet those mistakes, in our current legal system and our modern society, require us to spend the best years of our lives in a cage, followed by judgment and stigma that lasts however many years we have left.

We have done the time and we know what we did to deserve it, and we don't want to do it again.

And yet same as those of us addicted to food and laziness can be thrown right back into our old unhealthy cycles after suffering enough shame at the hands and eyes and hearts of judgmental others, the ex-cons I know feel chased every day by the ghosts of their mistakes. We are taunted by them every time someone asks about the gaps in our résumés and given judgmental looks, and from those who walk away from us on the sidewalk a little too quickly. These all trigger a desire for those old addictions. We know they are mistakes, but feel powerless to stop ourselves from committing those mistakes nonetheless, because in the mistake there is an old, familiar comfort, a sort of shelter from the way the world hurts us, not unlike when we were children and our parents hugged us.

Bad food. Booze. Dope. Getting a key neck-deep in the crack game. We are all different, but we all also have the same human brain, one so easily wired to run according to different little addictions.

‖‖‖‖‖‖

Second, the inspirational: I am not all that different from you.
  I'm still addicted to all kinds of things.
  It's just that now, I'm addicted to things that are healthy.
  Yeah, it was hard. But I know it's possible because I've done it.
  Now I am free.
  I just had to do the time.

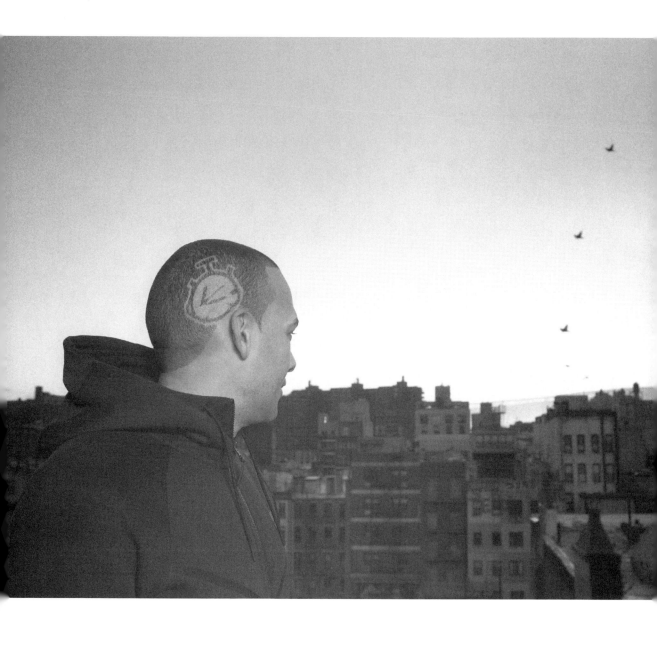

About the Authors

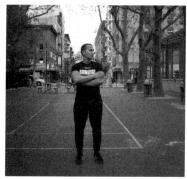

COSS MARTE is the owner and creator of ConBody, a growing gym and fitness business based on bodyweight and inspired by prison workouts. He was a Lower East Side drug dealer running his own crew and making bank before he turned his life around and became a legal entrepreneur committed to helping others get healthy and breaking down stereotypes to help other ex-cons like himself have a second chance at life.

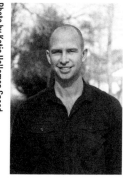

BRANDON SNEED is a writer-at-large for Bleacher Report's *B/R Mag*, where his story "I'm Not the Lone Wolf" was a finalist for the 2017 Livingston Award for best writers under thirty-five. He's also the author of three previous books, including *Head in the Game*, the story of his global quest to fix a fracturing mind that wrecked his baseball career and threatened to take the rest of his life with it. He blogs at brandonsneed.com. He lives in Greenville, North Carolina, with his wife and their two little boys.